REAL TALK REAL WOMEN

REAL TALK
REAL WOMEN

100 LIFE LESSONS FROM THE MOST
INSPIRATIONAL WOMEN IN HEALTH & FITNESS

MIRIAM KHALLADI

LIFECHANGE PRESS

AMSTERDAM

Copyright © 2013-2014 Miriam Khalladi

Published by LifeChange Press
http://www.lifechange.io

Always wanted to write and publish your own book?
Reach out to us via publish@lifechange.io

All rights reserved.

ISBN 10: 0991343506
ISBN 13: 978-0-9913435-0-8

Contents

Foreword by Tosca Reno	16
Introduction by Miriam Khalladi	18

VOLUME I - LOVE YOURSELF   21

Happy Girls Are The Prettiest	
by Mindy Ambrose	22
Be True to You	
by Dr. Catherine Divingian	26
Get Body Confidence Beautiful	
by Jennifer Ettinger	29
Believe in Yourself	
by Jill Gardner	32
Cultivating Healthy Self Esteem	
by Bry Jensen	34
Tap Into Your Greatness by Being Your Own Guru	
by Chivon John	39
It All Starts With You	
by Kelly Knox	43
The Power of Self Love	
by Dashama	46
Free Yourself	
by Bianca Lupo	50
Outer Beauty, Inner Beauty & Self Love	
by Laura Marie	53
Top 10 Tips on Living a Better Life	
by Nicole Moneer	58

The Two Women
by Rachel Elizabeth Murray — 60

The Awareness & Manifestation of Ego
by Karen Pang — 64

These 4 Words Could Change Your Life
by Donna Richards and Tora Cullip — 68

You Are Your Own 24/7
by Kristi Tauti — 72

The Tale of "The Barbell Pickup"
by Erica Willick — 76

VOLUME II - NEVER GIVE UP — 81

Fitness Saved Our Lives; Two Sister's Journey
by Elizabeth Aguilera & Morgan Wehmer — 82

The Three C's of Fitness Success
by Christine Anderson — 89

Fear of Failure
by Robyn Baldwin — 93

Overcoming Obstacles to Achieve Your Goals & Dreams
by Amy Bella — 99

Unbreakable
by Carla Maria Cadotte — 102

Nothing Comes Easy... But The Grind is Worth it
by Heidi Cannon — 111

How to Rise From The Ashes
by Phoenix Carnevale — 116

Katie's Journey to Happiness & Health
by Katie Cates — 120

Passion is Everything	
by Lori & Michelle Corso	124
Don't Tell Me I Can't	
by Dr. AnnMaria De Mars	128
Finding Your Inner Strength	
by Karen Gallagher	133
Female Perseverance	
by Liz Gaspari	138
Never Give Up	
by Nikki Giavasis	146
Stronger Than Yesterday	
by Stacey Goldberg	152
How to Turn a Setback into a Comeback	
by Ryall Graber	156
Why Didn't I Die?	
by Danny-J Johnson	163
Preserving Perseverance	
by Karen Kennedy	167
Dream Weaver	
by Sharzad Kiadeh	172
Never Give Up	
by Angelique Kronebusch	176
Living With Epilepsy	
by Jenny LaBaw	180
Persistence & Hard Work Always Pays Off	
by Tammy & Lyssie Lakatos	185
Healthy Mind, Healthy Body	
by Agostina Laneri	188

Clean & Bright Perspective	
by Theresa Jenn Lopetrone	191
Making Life Happen	
by Amy Markham	194
Fit Mama is Pregnant Again	
by Christie Nix	204
Empowering Women Worldwide	
by Elisabeth Nuesser	207
Finding Your Passion & Living Your Dreams	
by Shannon Petralito	211
My Life is a Progression, Not Perfect	
by Jessi Piha	216
A New Perspective; A New Stage	
by Lacey Pruett	220
I Crashed Into My New Life	
by Abigail Rich	225
Never Say "I Wish"... Make it Happen	
by Katie Rowlett	229
Having Faith in Your Surroundings	
by Jill Rudison	232
Get Out of Your Own Way	
by Cassandra Sawyer	239
Success Starts with Happiness	
by Andrea Smith	243
Life is Full of Detours	
by Nikki Stelzer	248
The Road to Recovery	
by Amy von Rummelhoff	252

Hard Work, Passion & Perseverance
by Jen Wenk   257

Finding Your Passion is Everyone's Quest in Life
by Shannan Yorton Penna   262

VOLUME III - ACHIEVE SUCCESS   267

The Power of Positive Thinking
by Victoria Adelus   268

5 Steps to Making Your Dreams Come True
by Bex Borucki   272

The Fitness Journey of Kelsey Byers
by Kelsey Byers   279

The Power of Choice
by Jacqueline Carly   282

Finding My Delicious Passion
by Tess Challis   287

Failure - The Greatest Secret to Success
by Diana Chaloux-LaCerte   292

Soul Awakening
by Rosie Chee   298

Creating Your Own Future
by Joanne Lee Cornish   301

Achieving Success
by Connie Garner   306

Secrets to Having a Mind Over the Matter
by Hilary Hagner   312

You Make Your Own Luck
by Natalie Jill   316

Follow Your Heart	
by Natasha Jonas	319
Becoming a Better Version of Me	
by Christine Keefer	321
Tough Love on Negativity	
by Kimber Kiefer	325
The 7 Lessons That Made Me a Champion	
by Julie Kitchen	330
Believe	
by Noora Kuusivuori	334
My Life is a Journey	
by Nicole G. Leier	338
Taking a Chance	
by Fatima Leite Kusch	340
Finding Your Passion	
by Amy Mac	343
Dreaming Big	
by Bridget McManus	348
Creating the Life You Love	
by Lindy Olsen	353
Rewriting the Story of Your Life	
by Marzia Prince	359
Achieving Success as a Figure Competitor	
by Louise Rogers	363
Putting the Love in Glove	
by Hedda Royce	367
Stay Driven & Focus on Your Dreams & Goals	
by Heather Shanholtz	370

Empowering Women
by Jana Stewart   373

Writing Contracts to Lifting Weights
by Tiffany Upshaw   377

Acknowledge Your Past, Embrace Your Future
by Deanna Wilson   381

What is Success? How is it Measured?
by Jenn Zerling   386

VOLUME IV - FIND BALANCE   391

Motherhood
by Alli Breen   392

Trust in the Process
by Rita Catolino   395

Finding Balance & Loving Yourself
by Kattie Fleece   398

My Life, My Puzzle
by Rose Gracie   401

How to Release Your Inner Zen
by Tara Milhem   406

Blessed
by Mary Schmitt   409

Superwoman; Fact or Fiction?
by Nicole Sims   412

Start; Healthy Lifestyle with Balance
by Dionne Sinclair   415

Who Are You Doing This For?
by Gaby Sink   419

You Can Have Your Cake & Eat it Too
by Abi Christine Woodcock   422

From Frumpy Mom to Buff Mom
by Stephanie Woods   425

VOLUME V - MAKE A DIFFERENCE   435

Creating Love in Every Day
by Kyla Gagnon   436

Find Your Inspiration
by Jessica Jessie   440

Making a Difference in the World
by Laura London   443

Never Give Up, Speak Out Loud
by Lindsey Meyer   446

Finding Fulfillment by Sharing Energy
by Heather Nicholds   453

Inspire People
by Valerie Solomon   456

About Miriam Khalladi   460

There's More!   461

Praise

"What an innovative thought, to look at female athletes as whole people - and go beyond the sound bytes and feel good personal interest features to look into their lives and lessons learned."
- Dr. AnnMaria De Mars

"It's wonderful to have all these fabulous empowering women speaking about their lives, goals, desires, tough times, passions and more and I'm so proud to be a part of it. It's a beautiful way to help others needing encouragement or, those trying to find their way in life. We all need those to look up to and towards for guidance as we all can learn from others. Thank you Miriam for putting us all together in such an amazing way! You are superb!"
- Shannan Yorton Penna

"What Miriam is doing is more than just creating a book. She is starting a movement. Women today struggle with so many issues when it comes to self-esteem, success, motivation, balance, etc. If more women teamed up like this to inspire and support one another, it could yield some truly powerful changes in society."
- Bianca Lupo

"I appreciate Miriam taking the time to spotlight the power, beauty, and strength that women embody. There is nothing more powerful to me than to see women helping other women by lifting them higher and supporting them."
- Kelly Knox

"Thanks so much Miriam for creating an avenue for many amazing women to share their inspiring stories with others. I am truly honoured to be included."

- Fatima Leite Kusch

"Health and fitness is often viewed two dimensionally; diet and training... When in reality the topic goes much deeper. Real Talk Real Women gives people the chance to see that we all struggle and conquer the same the things. I think this book is going to help a lot of women."

- Mary Schmitt

"Today's methods of conversation and the general media don't always give the entire story. Rather than having only the highlight reel, I'm grateful for Miriam's vision to share authentic stories from real-life women and real-life journeys."

- Lacey Pruett

"Miriam is in the process of helping spread the word of love, health and fitness with the help of top athletes and speakers in the industry!! What a woman to make this all happen!! Never let your fears deter you from achieving success!"

- Rita Catolino

"What an honor to be a part of such an amazing group of inspirational women and a project that is like no other done before. Thank you Miriam for the opportunity and for putting this together for others to get inspired as well. You are changing lives with this book."

- Noora Kuusivuori

Foreword by Tosca Reno

The decision to make change never comes lightly or easily. Most of us struggle to get to that point and then struggle yet again to embark on the path to change. All of us, myself included, need tools to help us along the way particularly because a great deal of support is required in the early stages.

How many of us have started, stopped, fallen, started and then given up altogether? If we are provided with powerful examples of women who have persevered throughout their journey we have a better chance to succeed ourselves.

By far and away the most effective tools include inspirational stories and the life lessons learned by those who have gone before us. Where would we be if we had not watched Martina Navratilova overcome personal struggle only to later become one of the most renowned female tennis players in the world.

Miriam's book, Real Talk, Real Woman, captures the real life stories of women who have embraced the call to change, answered it bravely if not sometimes blindly, faltered occasionally and ultimately succeeded.

The pages of this book share stories abundant with courage, determination and yes, even hardship. This is no valentine. This is a real woman's book to help other real women achieve their best selves.

Turn the pages slowly, absorbing this wealth of power. Take it in. Use it for your life. The power is now in your hands to change your life, for the better.

I am proud to be one of these women who have overcome much and can still find ample room to be grateful.

I am grateful to Miriam for this book.

I am grateful to you for reading it.

Much luck and strength on the way.

Tosca Reno

Tosca Reno is the New York Times best-selling author of Your Best Body Now and the Eat-Clean Diet® series, which has sold more than two million copies worldwide. She is one of the leading North American health and wellness experts fighting the battle against obesity. Tosca has a B.Sc., B.Ed. and is a certified Nutritional Therapy Practitioner (NTP).

Introduction by Miriam Khalladi

I was just a nobody.

At least that's what I thought just a little less than a year ago when we came up with the idea of "Real Talk Real Women" - a platform to inspire women across the globe to live healthier and happier lives.

"Why would any of these amazing women even agree to be interviewed by me?", "And what if they would, I'm shy and not used to speaking English.", "What if I freeze and don't know what to say?".

Negative self-talk. Doubt. Something many of us women will recognize as familiar. But at the same time I was curious. I wanted to know the real stories behind these women. Many of them were primarily portrayed for their beauty or athletic performances, but I knew there was more to it than that.

I was right.

As I interviewed well over a 100 women and listened to them share their lessons around self-love, never giving up, achieving success, finding balance and making a difference in the world - I realized that these interviews were just the beginning.

What you hold in your hands now is the culmination of our work this far.

As I read and then re-read the pages ahead I realized that nothing I could possibly write here would do justice to what is to come in the one hundred chapters ahead and while my name is on the cover, this is really their book.

So here's to the 105 amazing women from all over the world who have opened up their hearts and souls to make this all possible.

On top of that, I still can't believe that Tosca Reno wrote the foreword. When I met her in Las Vegas earlier this year she told me that she believes: "Everybody deserves a chance." - and I couldn't agree more.

All of these women deserve a chance to be heard. To be seen as real women. And I've made it my mission to help their voices be heard in a greater way. First through the on-going interview series and now through this book.

While we've compiled it with the utmost care, we've intentionally kept the chapters as they were, so that the authenticity and true voice of the authors shines through. Note that many of them (myself included) are not professional writers, so bare with us if you run into small mistakes.

And on this journey of mine, I realized something. I'm not a nobody. As you find yourself touched by the words ahead, what will you realize? Take a moment to reach out to our coauthors to let them know. I know they will appreciate hearing from you. You can find all of their details on the profile pages linked from each chapter.

Now, grab a notepad and a box of tissues and get ready to be touched and to be inspired as you go through these pages full of life changing wisdom.

Lots of love from Amsterdam,

Miriam Khalladi

P.S. We're constantly working on new projects to inspire people to lead healthier and happier lives. I'd like to invite you to join my free VIP list so that you don't miss out on new projects, the latest interviews full of inspirational wisdom and fantastic articles by our expert community! You can get on the list via www.rtrw.me/viplist

VOLUME I - LOVE YOURSELF

Happy Girls Are The Prettiest
by Mindy Ambrose

According to Audrey Hepburn, "Happy girls are the prettiest." I love this statement. It wasn't long ago that I didn't believe I could be classified as a pretty girl. It sounds strange now, but it took time for me to be able to say, "I'm a fitness model" out loud, without being apologetic. "Pretty" means something different to every person I've met. So why did I live for did I have such hang-ups over this word? It is just a word, but I feel as women, we give too much power to the masses' idea of prettiness. Is there a universal standard for prettiness? Of course there isn't. These days I feel pretty, even on my sweatiest, "no makeup" days -- hiking in the mountains with my nose running down my chin and cheeks flushed red and white. But, achieving this level of self-love was a three-year process, and I'm still fine tuning it.

I didn't see that there was something missing from my presumably confident self until I was training for my first physique competition in 2011. It seemed like everyone in my life was all of a sudden calling me a fitness model. I dreaded introductions from friends at parties, "This is my friend Mindy. She's a fitness model." I'd reply, "No. I'm an athlete. I'm not a model." I knew I wanted to take my stage goals far and I knew I wanted to be a big part of the health and fitness scene, but... a model? During these early months of competition prep, I had a hefty amount of confidence to build if I was going to prepare for opportunities as a motivational public figure. Knowing this didn't make the process any easier. I was still terrified that someone would point fingers at me for not looking like a real model once I was in the public eye. It sounds sad and negative, but we all have silly fears like these. We form fears based on unfounded rules we make up in our heads. Am I right? The truth is,

I was a generally confident and fearless person until this new chapter in my life began. This new identity was the ultimate test that exposed me for not fully loving myself like I thought I did.

I'm full of passion and possess gifts that not just anyone has; yet for a talented and intelligent woman, suddenly I was showing signs of a crazy and nonsensical self-image. I can't pinpoint where this struggle stemmed from. I'm sure experts would say it came from environmental factors like playing with Barbie dolls or watching TV shows centered around "beautiful" people. Perhaps it was the result of the many kids who had called me ugly in earlier years. (It seems like I've been called stunning as many times as I've been called ugly, which drove me bananas for a good 15 years). I think it was the first time I heard modeling terms like "commercial appeal" and "marketable look" when I blacklisted myself as a potential pretty girl. I don't have that commercial look that's commonly sought after in the modeling industry. So, I had to force myself to see that self-love comes from validation within me -- not from external sources like people or magazines. If external sources think I'm the cat's meow, that's a bonus, but they won't see it if I don't see it first.

I've always valued thick skin and fearlessness, so to force myself to gain some stage presence and get over my inhibitions (and hatred for smiling on demand,) I entered small bikini contests in my hometown. I braved all sorts of challenges in a matter of weeks, and was reaping rewards while doing it. I even won a competition to be the next professional ring girl at boxing events. Let me tell you, nothing fast-tracks confidence more effectively than standing in a bikini on stage next to girls who are 10 years younger, and lighting the room on fire. I was building confidence by simply practicing it and was earning some fans along the way. Most importantly, I was proud of myself for having guts and taking risks, and genuinely liked who I was becoming. No type of therapy compares to accomplishing heavy and intimidating goals. At this time I was making a shift from relying on external validation, to finally creating my own terms of validation. As I approached that first fitness competition I was planning to create a Facebook Page to build a following of like-minded women. I had the silly notion that I had to win a trophy in my competition before being worthy of publicly calling myself an athlete. I wasn't willing to welcome opportunities that came along with being a competitor (like modeling,) unless I could hide behind some credibility like a solid placing in a competitive show. I placed 5th in my category -- no medal or trophy. It was a great learning experience but to me no trophy meant "not a real athlete yet and absolutely not a fitness model." I'm embarrassed to say the old me didn't take the plunge into the public eye on her own. She practically had to be hog-tied, carried, and thrown in, to see what she was made of.

It was my partner Jason who then challenged me on the piles of self-doubt that had been oozing out my ears for months. He had watched me grow from a girl who wouldn't smile with her teeth showing; into someone who could at least fool an audience into believing she wasn't nervous. He didn't see why this rising star was terrified of going public with her new image and accomplishments. He refused to let me hold myself back any longer. He promised me for every one negative remark I may receive; I'd experience thousands of positive ones. With this, I begrudgingly launched my Facebook Page right after my first show. He was right! Nothing felt better than showing the world my real self, with conviction. This is something I want every woman with a dream to realize. It's especially vulnerable taking on goals where we know we will be publicly scrutinized. But, a ratio of one thousand fans for every one Negative Nellie is a pretty encouraging. Don't hold yourselves back from excellence. Every week I pinch myself, receiving compliments on my smile – that same smile that for over a decade had to be dragged out of me against my will.

Today I celebrate what sets me apart from other models. I accept having my dad's ears, Grandfather's cheeks, and my nana's ultra-fair skin. I do get rejected from opportunities. I do encounter cruel comments about my appearance on social media outlets... and... now watch those comments roll off my back. I'm Mindy Ambrose, pro-level competitive athlete, published writer and model, and public figure. It was a three-year uncomfortable process to self-acceptance as I grew into these titles, but I finally made it and I love myself more each day.

Mindy Ambrose

I'm a pro-level Canadian competitive fitness model, bodybuilding judge, published model and lifestyle writer. I'm known for encouraging others to not let age or insecurities hold them back from achieving their goals.

Be True to You
by Dr. Catherine Divingian

Lights. Cameras. Fame.

There's a part of all of us that craves the glamorous life of celebrity. We see them popping champagne corks, traveling in luxury, dining and shopping at the finest establishments, being waited on hand and foot, and having raving fans fawning over them. Who doesn't want to live in the illusion of being a queen, ruling the world?

And who isn't tired of being shuttled around where she doesn't want to go, being part of the cattle call in coach class when she flies, and banging her head against the glass ceiling at work? It's so tempting sometimes to just give it up and run away to join the proverbial circus.

What's really at the heart of the matter? Is it that you are actually craving a life of significance? Do you want to feel like you made a mark that will be remembered when you are long gone?

The big question is, how much of you are you willing to part with to become someone that is perceived as "important"? Would you pose nude, sleep with the casting director, take a few dollars from the office cash fund, or in any other way compromise your values? It's easy when you're not in a difficult situation to say that you would never be willing to make concessions. But when your back is against the wall and all of the things that you think that you crave are dangled before your eyes, what would you truly do?

I thought that I was an oak, impervious to temptation that would lead me to compromise. My stance on modeling was that I would not pose nude; nor would I even do an "implied" nude. My brand was based on professionalism, and I had strict limits. However, I found myself in front of a camera with another model in a beautiful bucolic setting with no one but the two of us and a very tricky photographer; I started posing in an increasingly sexy, risqué manner. It was starting to push my discomfort zone; yet I kept taking direction, the vision of fame and fortune that would result from the project dancing in my head.

But when the other model disappeared for a while and returned with her dress draped in front of her nude body, I knew that I was in trouble. The photographer was expecting the same from me. I called an end to the shoot. My photos were scrapped; and the photographer decided that a good, sound berating was necessary. I fled the shoot, disgraced and shaken to the core.

The problem was that I allowed the photographer to dictate terms for too long. I had lost the sense of who I was, and conveniently forgot what I stood for. Mulling over this event, I determined that it served as an important lesson that I must teach other women; and that this topic is the very heart of what it means to be truly self-confident.

The key is that you must know yourself. You need to have the courage to stand up for that truth, regardless of the cost. You will have to risk rejection and not getting what you want as easily as you hoped.

I was fortunate to have escaped with minimal damage. As the faculty advisor for Students in Free Enterprise, I headed up a project to help women from Nepal escape a life of slavery. Young women are often susceptible to wanting to believe promises of a better life and marriage to a wealthy man; and finding themselves lured into the hopeless situation of human trafficking. The Nepali Rescue Project helped raise funds to rescue women from slavery, and assist them with setting up honorable micro-entrepreneurial ventures. These survivors were able to provide a better standard of living for themselves and their families, and could finally hold their heads high with the first modicum of self-confidence they may have ever known. This was an extreme example; yet it happens to hundreds of thousands of women every year when they feel trapped and want an easy way out. It is the reality of the world for those that desire significance; but don't know how to achieve it.

This means that it is vital to be able to know the answer to the question, "What does significance mean to me?" Viktor Frankl, the survivor of a Nazi concentration camp asked that very question during the most frightening circumstances. His answer was that every moment that we are alive, we are significant.

This is tough for us to fully grasp Frankl's message when we feel invisible and are blinded by stars in our eyes. It's particularly the case when the wolves in sheep's clothing are not evident; and we see others who seem to be blessed with more passion and fortune than we are.

At each moment, we are given choices. When we honor who we truly are, we are living our Truth. It comes from being responsible for each moment, knowing ourselves, taking charge of the decisions, and moving forward to claim the lives we were meant to live. Perhaps you won't get to taste Dom Perignon and be draped in diamonds; but will your children, friends, or partner care? What will your legacy be? To be the envy of the world? Or to have mattered to those whose lives you touched, and known as a woman who lived life on her terms?

Hundreds of years ago, Shakespeare penned the maxim that holds to this day, "To thine own self be true." Treat yourself and your life as a gift, and you will find your significance.

Dr. Catherine Divingian

I'm an accomplished scientist, professor, author, speaker, athlete and wellness expert helping women achieve a fierce mind, powerful beauty.

Get Body Confidence Beautiful
by Jennifer Ettinger

"Why do we strive for perfection when we should strive to be whole"
– Jane Fonda

We all have seen her walk into a room, with her flowing hair, glowing skin and a radiant smile that takes over the room. I call this the "goddess glow," A beauty that is simply not captured in a bottle. It is called CONFIDENCE. The definition of confidence, according to the Oxford dictionary is "a feeling of self-assurance arising from an appreciation of one's own abilities or qualities"

How you view your body is the foundation as to how you feel about yourself. So many women cause undue stress as to how they should look vs. how they think they should look.

Getting body confidence is critical to one's success! Here are some tips to "reframe" your thinking of your current "goddess" body!

Your body is a beautiful gift. It allows you to live life to its fullest; emotionally and physically. It should be viewed as your best friend. Focus on what you enjoy about your body. Is it beautiful eyes, a dimple, a big smile? Be proud of your goddess assets!

Take the one feature you think is your BEST asset and great a daily mantra. For example, if it is your smile, you can say the following: I love my smile for it brings happiness into my life and to others. Then write a list of positive things about yourself! "I embrace my goddess shape. I will fuel my body with beauty boosting foods"

Understand that body image and self-esteem are different! How you look today is not how you are destined to be! Think of your current body and your health as a baseline to where you want to go and transform into.

Daily activity can make profound change in your life and help you reach your goals. Make the goal(s) specific. An example is: I will walk 3 times this week for a half hour vs. I will start walking. Keep a journal of your activity, food daily mantras and mood, to serve as a blueprint for your lifestyle changes.

Eat clean food and water, although we all are aware we should do this, many of us do not find the time to plan out our meals. Taking the time will make a profound effect on your body image. Fueling your body with the right nutrients will nourish the cells, and give you a newfound sense of energy, and healthy skin, nails and teeth. You will begin to shift your craving away from processed foods to reaching for a healthy alternative. As for your water, take our weight in pounds, and divide by 2. That is how many daily ounces of water you should be consuming.

Next, draw a line drawing picture of your body. Circle the areas that are "areas of concern." Ask yourself, the following questions. Are your concerns of BODY (food/exercise needed) or of MINDSET (being hard on yourself) Write in a journal your concerns and see if it aids you if finding a resolution. Often we KNOW what to do we just need to begin the journey.

Mirror, mirror on the wall, who is the fairest Goddess of all! Look into the mirror and OWN your reflection! Use this as a tool to measure your success! Each day is a stepping stone to your success, embrace the journey. This can be challenging. I encourage you to look yourself in the eyes and say, I LOVE .. (Your name) in the mirror. Work up to one minute a day, for ultimate self-love and acceptance!

You are whom you surround yourself with! Surround yourself with positive people of like minds! Ditch the one who wants to sabotage your success! Maybe it is time for a friend detox; release those who hinder you from being successful with a healthy lifestyle change. Embrace positive people who will LIFT you to new heights.

Lastly, skinny does not mean healthy! We hold celebrities on a podium of "beauty", but the reality is many are very unhealthy and unhappy! Be aware but do not compare. Focus on YOU!

Remember, "Body awareness leads to body confidence which resonates a body beautiful".

Jennifer Ettinger

I'm a best selling author. National brand ambassador for New Balance. TV show host & co-producer. Keynote speaker. Fitness & style expert.

Believe in Yourself
by Jill Gardner

I am a health & fitness lover. My friends know me as JillyG. I am currently studying for my ISSA PT Cert. I am a Radiologic Technologist & a Quest Nutrition Athlete. Born & raised in beautiful St. Augustine, FL. Growing up I was very active. I was involved in gymnastics, Winterguard & soccer. When I graduated high school I was introduced to the gym & weight lifting but didn't really fall in love with it until I got the nutrition part down! That's when the results came!

My childhood was far from happy & pleasant. You see I grew up with a sister that was verbally abusive. Every time I would turn around all I heard was you're fat, ugly, stupid & worthless. I couldn't understand why someone I looked up to. Someone that I loved would say such awful things. As we grew older & farther apart I would catch myself repeating those awful words to myself. Even though I knew it was far from the truth (having grown up with wonderful loving parents) part of me believed it. Part of me felt like if that's what my own sister thought of me there must be some truth to it. All throughout my 20's I was pretty self-destructive. I had developed an eating disorder as a teenager, which thankfully I have overcome. I was always so kind to others but when it came to myself there was no self-love, no self worth...

In my late 20's I remember tearing my closet apart looking for something to wear for a night out with friends. I hated who I saw in the mirror. I was so unhappy with myself. I spent way too many late nights out partying and eating terrible food. I was always hiding half of my body behind someone in pictures. I knew something had to change so the journey began.. After researching online & reading through fitness magazines I picked up a copy of The Eat-Clean Diet. I began to understand the importance of good food choices. I spent countless hours in the grocery store studying food labels. The weight started coming off slowly and I felt better than I ever had in my entire life. For once I felt comfortable in my own skin. I devoted a lot of time to my health & my happiness. I made it a priority to work on my mental health as well as my physical health.

Once I started taking weight training seriously it wasn't so much of a dreaded chore it had become an extremely healthy outlet. Something that I looked forward to every single day. A healthy happy place where I could release, let my guard down & just be me. I find great comfort in the weight room. The sound & the smell of the iron gets me pumped up! & being able to curl as much as some of the guys is very empowering! There's a quote that I now live by..

"The good Lord gave you a body that can stand most anything, it's your mind you have to convince" - Vince Lombardi

On days that I'm struggling I repeat this to myself over & over & just push through. Whether it's in the gym or in my personal/work life I keep this with me. It's amazing how our thoughts can affect us! You HAVE to believe in yourself!

Sure we all have good & bad days but knowing that I have inspired others & that I continue to do so pushes me to do better & be better! You have to lead by example! We have come so far with social media, which gives a great platform to share my journey, & continue to help improve the lives of others. It is truly humbling.

Jill Gardner
I'm a Health & Fitness lover. Quest Nutrition Athlete. RT (R).
Currently studying for my ISSA PT Cert.

Cultivating Healthy Self Esteem
by Bry Jensen

"Be who [you are meant] to be, and you will set the world on fire."
– St. Catherine of Siena

The world is what we make of it, and in turn, what we make of ourselves. There is a tremendous power that lies within us all, that determines whether we will succeed or fail, whether we will be joyful or miserable – and it is called self-esteem. This chapter will divulge my reflections on the impact and power of self-esteem, and how to best cultivate a healthy sense of self-esteem to ensure a lifetime of success and happiness.

Defined, self-esteem is the emotional evaluation of an individual's sense of worth that dictates the attitude and judgments made towards the self. Self esteem is not an organic entity, we do not come pre-programmed with how we feel about ourselves, nor can we be measured by any particular pre-existing scale; rather self esteem is an intensely personalized perspective shaped by our thoughts, actions, environment, and circumstances. It is the internalized thoughts and feelings that even in its essence can be different between every individual, with the ultimate outcome of feeling good about who we are. Why is this so critical to every aspect of our lives? It is because self worth is the internal compass we use to navigate our world and how we perceive our value; self-esteem dictates how we feel about the way other people treat us, what we believe we deserve, and what we will tolerate when it comes to the health of our emotional, physical and spiritual selves, the parts of the whole of our person. Self-esteem shapes our personal expectations, and how strongly we believe in our abilities and strengths.

Having a healthy sense of self esteem is the foundation of confidence, which allows us to be who we are, express who we are, and to enjoy doing it! It is the driving force that urges us to pursue goals, persevere in them because we believe we are capable of greatness. It encourages us to walk away from destructive situations, because healthy self-esteem allows for self-reflection and critical evaluation, without damaging our self-worth. The importance of healthy self-esteem is most exemplified in its absence; having low self-esteem can be one of the most detrimental obstacles to face in your life, as it can project an aura of negativity that can hinder our ability to feel good, to make smart decisions, or even to pursue our dreams. It can feel hopeless, impossible, as if you are drowning or caught in darkness without a way out. For this reason, cultivating a healthy sense of self-esteem is one of the most advantageous and beneficial personal skill sets you can acquire.

The most important step of cultivating your healthy self-esteem is to first discover who you are. Self-esteem and confidence can only exist in an environment of authenticity; pretending to be something or someone that you are not is a personal declaration that who you are is not desirable or worthy, and an indication of low self-esteem. Finding one's identity is not necessarily easy, nor is it a one-step process. It will take time, and it is okay to be confused about your identity, because developing your sense of self and personality is a growing and learning experience filled with ongoing changes. Therefore, being true to this explorative process is crucial to healthy self worth. One path to your true self is exploring your passions, to discover what activities and dreams inspire you to feel accomplished, and to investigate goals that test your boundaries. Locating aspects of your life where your passion shines will allow you, and your confidence to flourish.

To ensure the authenticity of your self-exploration, do not be afraid to embrace your quirks and flaws. Self-esteem is an honest power; it does not delude or deceive, and it will not give you the image of perfection. Instead, having a healthy self-esteem brings about the understanding that no one is perfect, everyone has flaws and struggles, and embracing that reality is a monumental step towards feeling good. It will be a strong reminder that though there may be aspects of yourself you feel self conscious about or may not entirely like, you are no less amazing. It is impossible to ignore these feelings; therefore the learning experience is to accept your flaws, your weaknesses and challenges, to work on them or to embrace things you are unable to change. With the right positive mindset, the character faults you perceive about yourself can be overcome, modified into strengths, or accepted as not as glaring as they may feel. Flaws and peculiar or unique quirks are a part of who you are, and should be loved and accepted as much as the parts of yourself that you are proud of.

Self-esteem is a social animal, and part of the journey towards confidence and self-assurance is finding a way to feel comfortable interacting with the world. Socialization has a huge impact on our self-esteem, and how we perceive our value to society. For this reason, do not be afraid to seek help from others while working on your self-esteem. Most importantly, surround yourself with positive people who will lift you up, rejoice in your accomplishments and support you and your goals, rather than bring you down or criticize your efforts. Seek out the people in your life that inspire you to be better, as your genuine, authentic self. Often, some of the most negative influences on our self esteem can be our closest kept company, and it may be difficult to distance yourself from negative people in your life, but being able to separate yourself from negativity will greatly enhance how you feel. In the company of people who boost your confidence and self-appreciation, it will quickly become apparent that positive social circles have magnetic qualities. Therefore, when you are working to build your sense of self worth, pay attention to the people who project a positive energy and willingness to support and give confidence, and draw them into your life. They will be your support network, folk you can rely upon for encouragement in your self-building goals. Furthermore, surrounding yourself with people who help your spirit flourish will make you a beacon for others who will be drawn you and your passions.

Creating a positive social atmosphere and support network is a milestone, yet it is equally as important to engage in positive individually driven experiences as well, such as taking time to explore and reflect. Individually driven experiences can be to do something that scares you, and to overcome the perceived hurdles holding you back. Being able to instigate experiences that enhance how you feel about yourself will reinforce the fact that a social group is not absolutely necessary to initiate healthy self esteem, rather they can be an added benefit. Individually driven experiences are thought provoking and reflective, to help reveal what areas of your life may need more work. For example, if you were to wake up each morning and tell yourself that you are a beautiful person with a genuine soul, a wonderful mind and a warm caring heart, and something about the statement does not feel comfortable, it is important to reflect on why you feel this way, and to develop new skills for dealing with your uncertainties.

Cultivating self-esteem is also the perfect environment for the creation of healthy habits, which will in turn reciprocate your efforts. Your body listens to the positivity of your mind, and adapts to perform better, just as a healthy body will encourage the mind towards positive thinking. This means taking care of yourself – eating and sleeping well, engaging in adequate exercise, and managing your stress is important in creating a physical atmosphere where your growing self esteem can flourish. Maintaining the lowest stress level possible will enhance your ability to master tasks, and facilitate healthy hormones for productive thinking. Treating your body right will result in a physical craving for further positive, healthy treatment and the mind is similar in that when you feed it with positivity, it will flourish and both demand and share more. Feed your mind with positivity by forging affirmative habits, such as writing down your successes and strengths, or rewarding yourself for your hard work with things or activities you enjoy doing. Building positive habits such as these will curb negativity-spreading habits such as gossiping or putting others down, for they will feel toxic in your emotional space. Negativity, and the sharing of it, will only destroy authentic self-esteem, and may also be harmful to others who also might be struggling with their self worth. In committing to habits of positive thinking, encouragement, and self-reflection, you will help shape and grow your self-esteem.

Finally, you can use this positive outlook and positive habits in all aspects of your life, including setting goals. Often, the desire to create and pursue a new goal is instigated by a level of dissatisfaction, or unhappiness with ourselves. However, the most successful and well-won goals are inspired by self-esteem – when we believe we are worthy and deserving of something great, our journeys are clearer, defined, and we are more capable of success. When goals are made in a positive mindset, we can, and will reach them. The journey to self-esteem can be a long and arduous path, but it is a trip worth traveling. With a healthy sense of self-esteem and confidence, there is nothing that you cannot do!

Bry Jensen
I'm a Magnum sponsored athlete, published fitness model, writer and ISSA certified personal trainer dedicated to inspiration, fitness and health.

Tap Into Your Greatness by Being Your Own Guru
by Chivon John

> "The greatest guru is your inner self.
> Truly he is the supreme teacher.
> He alone can take you to your goal and
> he alone meets you at the end of the road.
> Confide in him and you need no outer guru."
> - Nisargadatta Maharaj

86,400.

That is the number of seconds in one day. It's a significant number yet many will likely argue that it never feels like it is enough.

When we live in an age that encourages you to do it all, it's no wonder that we have nagging whispers of discontent that make us believe that we should DO and BE more. More often than not, we find ourselves on a quest looking for answers from others on how we can be at the top of our game, get more done, look better and feel whole.

But here's the fallacy with this cycle. When we seek out the knowledge of guru's to replace your own wisdom you'll always be in the habit of constantly looking outside of yourself for answers.

Don't get me wrong. The knowledge of your mentors or 'guru's is valuable. I consider myself to be a lifelong student and crave the chance to learn something new at any available opportunity. However, it's important to understand that the wisdom of our teachers should serve to inspire you to turn inward, instead of making you believe that we don't know enough to guide your own path.

Far too often we convince ourselves that we need degrees, certifications or certain life experience to bestow wisdom to others and especially ourselves. But this is a mindset that is rooted in scarcity and will always leave you feeling that you're never good enough.

If you've ever found yourself on a never-ending quest for answers, it's important to know that you're not alone. In Dr. Brene Brown's book The Gifts of Imperfection, she referred to this as the 'hustle for worthiness'.

When we fail to acknowledge what we have in the here and now, recognize our strengths and the trials that we have overcome, our soul will continue to remain emaciated. It will steadily starve in search of nourishment that can only be quenched by looking in the mirror and accepting the person that you see in the reflection.

If you only remember one thing, know this: You are enough.

When you spend your life stuck in the story of your circumstances it's impossible to see the beauty that exists within YOU.

I know it's not easy but your soul depends on it and you're worth the effort. After years of sweeping over my own emotions, I've learned that there is an immense power in acknowledging your feelings and internal wisdom. But there is an even greater strength that happens when you learn to use your story to heal yourself and empower others.

So, consider this your permission slip to stop waiting for the right guru to come along to answer your questions. You have permission to affirm that you are enough right now as you are and that you are the expert on your life!

It's time to stand on your story, tap into your inner guide and own your greatness!

Still not convinced that you can be your own Guru? Here are 3 inspired action challenges to reveal your inner wisdom:

1. **Turn your wounds into wisdom**

When we experience a setback it's easy to fall into the woe is me mantra or feel as if the odds are stacked against us. Oprah's powerful quote "turn your wounds into wisdom" is a powerful affirmation to empower us to identify the greater lessons through our tribulations. Think of all of the turbulent times in your life and write them down on a piece of paper. In a column beside each line item ask yourself, 'What can I learn from this?' or 'How will I become a better person through this experience?' Life presents us with teachable moments every day and even during difficult or sad times we can emerge stronger and wiser.

2. Acknowledge why you are awesome

Can you name at least 10 reasons why you are amazing? Grab a sheet of paper and write down 10 qualities about yourself that make you the amazing, unique and awesome person that you are. Don't feel bad if you struggle with this exercise. Phone up a friend or family member and have them help you by sharing what they love the most about you.

Allow this list to elevate you when you're feeling down and also empower you daily to know why you are the master of your life. As a bonus, identify the ways that you can share your special gifts with the world. Play to your strengths and acknowledge why you're special instead of focusing on your perceived weaknesses.

3. Practice gratitude daily

Take an oath of practicing gratitude. This can take the form of writing it down in a journal or creating a gratitude jar. Gratitude is a powerful practice because it allows us be present.

It forces us to slow down and demands that we travel through life awake instead of sleepwalking. There is no time to question or overthink when you think about why you're grateful.

The best part about practicing gratitude is that it allows you to banish your scarcity mindset and manifest more positivity into your life by focusing on what you have instead of what you don't.

Above all remember: You don't need to ask for permission to be who you are.

There will never be a right time. If you find yourself asking "Am I ready?" The answer is likely always NO, so do it anyway and your first choice of guru can be found in the mirror.

The strongest relationship in your life should be the one with yourself. It's not easy by any means but fight for you because you're worth the effort! People will come and go in your life but the one constant is that you'll always be with yourself. Love the one that you're with and stand up and own your greatness.

Chivon John

I'm a wellness advocate, communications strategist, writer and speaker. I'm passionate about inspiring people to put self-care at the top of their priority list and to learn how to be fully engaged in every moment.

It All Starts With You
by Kelly Knox

Although fitness was something that I stumbled upon, it has changed my life in so many ways. And I would love to share my journey with you. It all started for me after deciding that I wasn't happy or settled in my life. I married very young, and coupled with having a child at that time, I never really explored or investigated who I was or what I wanted out of life. I was just going with the flow, with no real direction or drive. I was tremendously in question of who I was and what I stood for. Looking back this was so evident even in the way I carried myself on a day-to-day basis. I wore sweat pants every day, paired with a ponytail and no make-up. I didn't take care of my body, my mind, my spirit, or my soul. I was more unsettled than I could ever put words on. That is when it hit me like a ton of bricks. I had been living a life that wasn't true to me and I had no idea who I was. There was something in me that did not want to live this way.

Something I like to describe as an "itch" to DO better and BE better. Although it took every little bit of strength and courage I had, I decided to act on it. Terrified of the unknown, but equally as uncomfortable with where I was sitting at the time, I contacted a therapist and my life hasn't been the same since. I explored things that were holding me back, wounds that needed to be healed, and pain that had to be addressed. By doing this I was able to be free and allow myself to grow, heal, and explore what I really wanted out of this wonderful journey we call life! There was a two-year period of time in which I cried almost every single day.

After all I was forced to look at things that I had chosen to ignore my entire life. Things that had caused me so much pain that I learned to shut myself off and become numb. Being unable to feel had become my coping mechanism and truthfully for a long period of time it served me well. It allowed me to survive certain circumstances without turning to drugs, alcohol or any other outside sources but unwinding this way of surviving was the most challenging task I have ever faced. I have always wished I was able to explain what kept me showing up to those appointments every Thursday despite how difficult they were but something in me wanted more out of life and although I considered quitting many times I am so thankful I never did.

I gained not only self-respect, but I learned to value myself as an individual person. I faced fears and began to break down my walls, and to heal many wounds that were holding me back from going after what I really wanted. For me, that was to be comfortable in my own skin and really learn to love, embrace, and embody who I am at my core without fear of disapproval from others. I wanted to live life by my own accord and do what feels good to ME, not anyone else.

I faced plenty of opposition along the way but I chose to stick my head down and do the work I had set out to do and decided not to omit pieces of me to make others comfortable. Not everyone in my life at that time is still there and that's ok with me and truthfully, very necessary. Not everyone is meant to be in your life forever. Some are there for a short time. Perhaps it's to teach you a lesson or to help you see what you want and don't want. What you're willing to accept and what you're not. It is ok to outgrow people. It's ok to have a life that's going in a different direction. Friends, family, and experiences are all part of your journey. They make you who you are and that's what makes you unique!

Never be afraid to ask for help. We are not super humans. We are real women, living real lives and dealing with real issues. It all starts with YOU! When you are healthy and happy you have the power to get exactly what it is you want out of life! Making the decision to invest in myself and in my future slowly began to give me a confidence to go after more and more and I promise it will do the same for you.

This journey started to spill over into all aspects of my life, and I began to slowly take care of myself physically. Adding fitness and healthy eating to my life has given me a confidence and a strength that I had never known, and will never take for granted. I had horrible eating habits and the last place you would ever find me was a gym! I was eating fast food and sugar all the time and had no real idea of how bad I was actually feeling until I started eating "clean".

I still enjoy indulging in those things on occasion, but they are no larger a part of my regular diet. I feel better, look better, and feel more confident when I am feeding my body what it needs and what it deserves which is proper nutrition. I have lost over 25 lbs. over the course of my journey as well as gaining a ton of love and value for myself. It's nice being able to slip right into a pair of jeans, (anyone who tells you it isn't, is lying), but at the end of the day for me it's about taking care of myself and teaching my daughter why it is important for her to do the same.

Fitting into clothes is just a bonus! There are ups, downs, highs and lows. Easy days and hard days, but that's the beauty of life. It's not the number of times you get knocked down, but how many times you stand back up! I said "No, thank you" to the hand I was dealt, and you can too! You get one shot at this like ladies! Just one and if you choose to do it right I am confident that once is enough!

Kelly Knox

I am the mother of a beautiful, ten year old little girl named Ava. I have gained an absolute passion for fitness, clean eating, and authentic living after deciding to change my life from the inside out.

The Power of Self Love by Dashama

Self love is fundamental to living a good life. Whether you strive to be successful in your career, to have positive supportive relationships or to create excellent health and live a long fulfilling life, everything improves when we learn to love ourselves unconditionally. In this chapter, "The Power of Self Love" I share with you my top self love tips and the direct and immediate effect they can have to improve every aspect of your life, if applied and practiced consistently.

Each of us is born a perfect miracle of life manifest as a result of an instantaneous and divinely appointed union of egg and sperm. The true journey begins for our soul, as we take our first breath and experience the first separation from our creator, who at that time is in form as our mother.

According to yogic philosophy, we then proceed to spend the remainder of our life seeking to return to that state of perfect connection with our source. The journey from that state of miraculous divine perfection to self-love and gratitude for this life is not always easy. Life throws us curve balls, challenges, obstacles and it is our opportunity each and every day to choose love.

Theoretically, it sounds easy: Just choose love. Love yourself and love everyone else and be happy, successful and blessed.

So, if life can be that simple and easy, why don't we all just do that? The answer exists in our subconscious mind.

As we begin to develop our consciousness, in childhood, every experience we encounter is stored in our subconscious mind, sometimes referred to as unconscious mind. This is where the roots of our self-loathing and low self-esteem are planted.

There are some powerful ways I have discovered you can get to the deepest and most stubborn roots to eradicate suffering and peel the layers to reveal your true self that is divine perfection manifest in physical form. It is my responsibility to share these with you, since our only true responsibility in this life is to be happy and when we find what can alleviate suffering to help others to be happy, it is the greatest gift to pass that along. As we alleviate our own misery and pain, we in effect alleviate all of the pain in the world.

1. Let go of ego desire and be true to yourself. Your body, mind, heart and soul work together in a magical way to guide you through this journey of life. When we block our own intuition by living in our ego desire, we create suffering and disconnect from our true self. As we let go of ego desire and allow divine will to flow freely through us, we have no other option other than happiness, which is our true nature.

2. Take time immediately and daily for metta meditation, which is a practice of loving kindness where you send love, peace and happiness out to all beings in the world. This sharing of unconditional love awakens the same unconditional love for your own self, as you are just one of the billions of others you are sending love to, and you will start to see yourself as interconnected to all beings, thus creating a field of love and support energetically from all beings and to all beings all the time.

3. Smile, laugh, play, yoga, move, swim, dance, sing, make love and eat raw chocolate. When you allow yourself to experience the pleasures of life, you remind your soul of the innocence and joy of living. This is very important, as mind, body and soul must be united often to maintain that perfect connection and the more often you make this connection, the stronger it gets and the better you will feel about yourself.

4. Make love daily. This is not a sexual proclamation, although if you are in a divine relationship, if you can make that a practice to unite daily with your beloved, in sacred union, by all means, do that! But what

I am referring to is to make love with life. You can experience the same level of orgasmic bliss in silent meditation as you can making love with a partner, and when you achieve that state of samadhi meditation, you can sustain the sensation much longer than when in union with another person. The key to this is not to become attached to the experience or sensation, however. You take that essence, the energy of love and divine connection, the feeling of aliveness, and carry it with you all the time, in every moment. You carry the vibration of love and you become loving kindness. This is a tantric practice and it can serve you infinitely as you journey through this life. Notice when you are not feeling that love vibration in your body, mind or heart and stop to release the negative or stuck energy that may be blocking the free flow of love. This is your daily practice and nothing is more important that it should prevent you from this practice.

5. Look in the mirror daily, and smile. Tell yourself all of the amazing things about yourself and when other people give you a compliment, thank them, believe them and allow that truth to permeate your conscious, into your own self limiting subconscious so you can release any and all negative thoughts, beliefs and emotions you may be carrying about yourself and others! When you carry negative beliefs and thoughts about yourself and others, it robs you of your joy and blocks the self love from flowing freely.

When you are able to be freed from these limiting beliefs, blocks and patterns, you are free. When you are free, you become like water fluid you are now responsible only to maintain that energy of self-love, pass it along to others and serve in every way you are able to. Be love, see love and goodness in others. Allow love into your life and trust that everything is unfolding in divine time. Let go of the past, don't focus on the future, live in the present and miracles will unfold for you every step of the journey.

Infinite blessings to you on your path.

Blessings and Love.

Namaste.

Dashama

I'm an International Yoga Teacher & Author and organize Teacher Trainings & Adventure Travel Transformation Retreats in Bali. I'm also the Producer of WeR1Race events.

Free Yourself
by Bianca Lupo

There was a time when I was ripped to shreds. I was 10% body fat at most. My muscles had muscles. I have to say, my body was very impressive. As a professional dancer and fitness professional, I received compliments constantly. My body helped to get me jobs and clients. People asked me my secret because they wanted to look the way I did. My secret was, that I was silently suffering while food and exercise controlled my whole life.

I trained every single day, sometimes twice a day. I brainwashed myself into thinking that I was a 'clean eater' when truthfully, food was my enemy. Social functions scared me since I couldn't plan my own menu. If I ordered a meal while out to eat and they messed up by not omitting things like cheese or oil, I would go into full panic mode until it was resolved. My issues with food went to such extremes; I would need all the pages in this book to share all the stories...

I see so many people striving to look like some variation of what I did during this time. But the truth is, I was restrictive, obsessive, and miserable. My priorities were completely bogus. I was missing out on so much of life because of my preoccupation with diet, fitness, and my body. I may have looked healthy, but I was so far from it.

In hindsight, I realize that I was obsessed with my physique because I felt completely empty on the inside, so I had to strive for perfection on the outside. I was living in denial of several painful childhood issues, and instead of dealing with them, distracted myself with things I could easily control and manipulate. I let my self-confidence fall victim not only to these issues, but the warped societal norms so many of us hold ourselves to. I wanted to feel accepted. Special. Loved. I was so completely unaware of how to give myself those feelings, that I strived for the external validation that I COULD be accepted, special, and loved. Searching for it that way is like a dog chasing its tail. The more you try, the farther you seem to get.

I am at a point now where I am physically much softer and ever so much happier. Fitness and nutrition have become a love and a passion rather than an unhealthy obsession or obligation. I have made it my life's work to help other people learn to develop healthy and loving relationships with themselves, food, and their bodies. The suffering and self-punishment in regards to food, health, and body image MUST end. If I can use my story to help and reach out to even just one person, then it was worth the struggle.

I have learned to accept who I am (although this truly is a never-ending process) and have grown to value myself for what I contribute to the world and those around me... not because I have perfect abs. If you die tomorrow, NO ONE in your eulogy will talk about your abs. No one will care how thin you were. Or how soft and shiny your hair was, how straight your teeth were, or the size of your hips. What will matter is WHO you were, and the impression you made on those around you.

Perfection is defined as "the condition, state, or quality of being free or as free as possible from all flaws or defects." If that is the case, then you are already perfect. Flaws and defects are self-imposed. You can choose not to succumb to the societal norms that our self-esteem perpetually falls victim to. If you redefine what "flaws" are... or more so, what they AREN'T, then you can free yourself of them. You can choose, right now, to be "perfect." Just like that. Go ahead... free yourself....

Live your life, enjoy these numbered days, and learn to love yourself however you are at this very moment. Strive to be the best you can be, and whatever that is, love it. No one gets out of life alive... you get one chance. There is so much love out there just waiting for you. And it all starts within.

Bianca Lupo

I'm a fitness/nutrition specialist, professional dancer, lover of life and all things wellness!

Outer Beauty, Inner Beauty & Self Love
by Laura Marie

"Beauty is not in the face; beauty is a light in the heart." - Kahlil Gibran
"Outer beauty attracts, but inner beauty captivates." - Kate Angell

Beauty is probably one of my favorite topics to talk about. There are those words which one enjoys hearing aloud and seeing written because it makes us feel all kind of emotions, you know, the kind that gives us goose bumps. Beauty does that for me, along with the word magic. Both of these words evoke a sense of dreaming for me, they take me to a parallel world, of imagination, colors, creativity, self-expression, light, purity and love.

We can all create beauty, with our words, with our thoughts, with our actions. The kind of Beauty I'm talking about is not limited to physical beauty and external attributes. Beauty comes from within and everybody can ignite beauty as soon as they're willing to take a ride into their heart and their soul.

Although part of my job is to help women lose weight and look their best, my main message has always been that a complete transformation has to form from the inside, out. External beauty is nothing without a beautiful light in your soul and without healthy self-love.

When Outer Beauty Meets Inner Beauty

Inner Beauty really is what makes us shine and sparkle. However, it is very important that women love themselves physically too - meaning loving their bodies and loving who they are in general.

It is not possible to be truly happy if you hate what you see everyday in the mirror. This causes very unhealthy self-talk, which can lead to all kinds of health and relationships issues. I've been through it when I was younger, and I know how painful self-hate is. Wanting to be anybody else but who you are is one of the most awful feelings on earth. Feeling ashamed of your body, and who you are, is truly hurtful and paralyzing. However, this tough experience with self-hate brought me to where I am today. Only through contrast can we give birth to new powerful desires such as wanting to become the best version of ourselves, physically, mentally and spiritually. This is what happened to me.

The thing is, you shouldn't want to change your physique in order to fit any society standards, or trend, but to really become the best representation of who YOU want to be, and of the image you want to project to the world, whatever that image is, as long as YOU like it and stay true to your SELF.

What Kind of Woman Do You Want To Be?

You have the right to want to look and feel beautiful. If you like to admire the beauty of a lion or a tiger, then why feel ashamed of wanting to express your own beauty? You are a piece of art! You are unique and have something special to bring to this world. Never be ashamed of wanting to shine and express beauty in your own ways.

I take care of myself physically – through eating foods of the highest vibrational quality (yes, food has a vibration, just like our thoughts and everything that exists on this planet) – and through regular exercise (strength training and cardiovascular training).

But I also give care a lot to my mind, by deliberately choosing positive thoughts over negative ones, by choosing very carefully the people that surround me and paying attention to where I put my focus on (always directed to what I do want and not what I fear or don't want). For my spirit, I meditate, and connect quite often to my inner guidance (intuitions), for this is the whisper of our soul. I have my inner world and I feel that's what makes me the most powerful in my life.

The more you flourish on the inside, the more this light will reflect on the outside. You may finally lose the weight you tried to lose for ages, and your body may even take another shape. In fact, that's literally what happened to me! My body totally changed, to a degree I could have never imagined possible. I am now who I want to be, and this is the most beautiful feeling ever.

Self Love

Self-love is the root from which everything grows. It impacts every single thing or person that is part of your life - and lack of self-love is the number one cause for most of our problems in life, if not all.

I would say that loving ourselves in a genuine, healthy, and respectful is one of the most difficult tasks we have to realize in life.

Yet, this one of the single most important lessons because the most powerful relationship we'll ever have is the relationship with ourselves.

I'm going to share with you a tool that I learned from a spiritual teacher (The Spiritual Catalyst: Teal Scott) which I find incredibly powerful. This technique is called "What Would Someone Who Loved Themselves Do?".

I want you to ask yourself this question, each time you want to do something or have to make a decision, even the most minor decision: "What would someone who loved themselves do?".

As this spiritual teacher describes it, the answer will come immediately, as a flash of intuition.

Your intuitions are your "higher-self" speaking to you, that part of you that knows much more than the thinking-mind.

Each time you're about to eat something, do something, or make a decision, once again, ask yourself "What would someone who loved themselves do?" and then have the courage to act on the answer, even if you don't understand it right away.

Know that everything is always part of a much bigger plan and that your higher-self always knows what to do for your highest good...

"The person in life that you will always be with the most, is yourself. Because even when you are with others, you are still with yourself, too! When you wake up in the morning, you are with yourself, laying in bed at night you are with yourself, walking down the street in the sunlight you are with yourself. What kind of person do you want to walk down the street with? What kind of person do you want to wake up in the morning with? What kind of person do you want to see at the end of the day before you fall asleep? Because that person is yourself, and it's your responsibility to be that person you want to be with. I know I want to spend my life with a person who knows how to let things go, who's not full of hate, who's able to smile and be carefree. So that's who I have to be."
- C. JoyBell C.

I once heard that bliss was « the sweetest nectar of life », and I agree on a profound level. Bliss is physical, emotional, spiritual, and mental happiness and this is the most delightful feeling on the planet... for this is when you are in complete alignment with who you truly are, and who you truly want to be.

Finding bliss is not always an easy quest, but for me, it is the most fascinating one. It requires a lot of courage, drive and passion, which a lot you encounter may not have, but I promise when you begin this quest, you'll begin the greatest journey of your life.

Love,

Laura Marie

I am a business owner, a writer, a life coach, a certified personal trainer and model. I inspire and help women to become the best version of themselves (physically, mentally and spiritually).

Top 10 Tips on Living a Better Life by Nicole Moneer

Here are my top 10 tips on living a better life:

1. It's not always about you. Stop reacting and escalating situations with loved ones or colleagues. Step back. Inhale deeply and slowly. Listen to others, be compassionate and validate the other person's feelings. Most people aren't complaining or nagging (even though it may come across that way), most people have hurt feelings that need to be expressed.

2. Stop putting your work and Internet before people. Those things will be around forever the important people in your life will not. Most people just wanted to be loved more. They want your time. They want your undivided attention. They want you to be a part of their life.

3. It's ok to say I can't. It's ok to say I'm not strong enough. It's ok to lean on other people. It's ok to be vulnerable. It wasn't until my Mom's death last year in 2012 that I finally did this. It feels good to let someone else take care of you. It feels good to let others know I'm human and I can't do it all. It feels good to let others love me and embrace me during some of my weakest life moments.

4. You'll survive. You always have and you always will. Everything may not happen how you want it. No matter how bad things get enjoy the life lesson and the strength you gain along the way.

5. Start looking in the mirror. Stop pointing the finger out. Work on yourself not other people and others things. Unhappiness is a disease. You always have the power to change and be happy. You can only change and better yourself, if you want to.

6. Tell your parents siblings spouse children significant other and closest friends how much you love them and appreciate them. Tell them

what you admire about them. Compliment them. Give them praise. If you can't say it write it in a card or an email. Then they'll have those awesome words forever to look at. My mom saved so many cards that my father brother & I gave her. She knew we loved her so much and we knew she appreciated us in return.

7. Practice saying I'm sorry. Be sincere. I used to suck at apologies. The better I got at them the better my life got.

8. Let people in. There are angels that walk this earth everyday. It sucks to put a wall up to everyone. I'm so glad I've let my walls down...slowly, to allow so many angels into my life. Two of my best friends Stacy & Staci to name a few...when I first met them I didn't trust them. I had my walls up for various reasons. They are two of the best people that entered my adult life. I'm so glad I let them in.

9. Reach out to people, with love. Most people may think you're just too busy for them or that you will reject them and say no if they each out to you.

10. Fall in love with yourself especially before adding another person to your life or falling in love with another. The single life can teach you exactly what you need as an individual and in a relationship. It can also teach you what you need to bring to a relationship and areas you need to work on in order to have a healthy successful relationship.

Nicole Moneer

I'm a NASM-CPT and Chek holistic lifestyle coach at life time fitness in Chicago, a bodybuilding.com athlete, an IFBB Bikini Pro & Olympian, as well as an internationally published fitness model & writer.

The Two Women
by Rachel Elizabeth Murray

*"The wise woman builds
her house,
but with her own hands
the foolish one tears
hers down."*

- - Proverbs 14:1 - -

I used to find it easy to convince myself that I was the first woman in this proverb. I was self-made! I was building my "house" and no one could stop me! In hindsight, I realize that for a long time, that attitude was just pride making up for the actual insecurity I had in my own unique purpose. I wasn't sure that what I had to offer in originality would 'make the cut' for the goals and dreams I had. In fact, I was actually the second woman, because while I believed I was pushing forward with sheer determination, I was so busy comparing myself to others who had gone before me, or to other women who are peers in my industry. Foolishly, I saw their accomplishments as things to out-do. While they succeeded doing certain things I wasn't doing, I found myself ignoring my own accomplishments, and wasted hour upon hour trying to do what they were doing, that I wasn't, assuming I needed to "do that too" (whatever that was) to be successful.

If you see life as objective, and every person as an architect, then the objective, or purpose, of life is to build your house. In this proverb, I was the second woman. Foolishly, I didn't see that no matter how much I strained, I would never realize my own purpose or reach my own potential by trying to copy and paste the lives of my peers and mentors into my own story. All that did was cultivate a competitive, jealous, aggressive, and toxic heart, which in turn seeped into other areas of my life in the form of gossip, envy, or even silence (for example, I'd simply avoid sharing comments or compliments that would encourage or 'edify' industry peers and mentors because I 'had to' have the 'advantage'). I'm gonna go out on a limb here and just say that those are not character traits you want when you're entire career goal is to inspire and empower the masses. Just saying. They are, however, symptoms of a very clouded perspective on life. I wasn't building my house. I was tearing it down.

Note: The problem isn't in emulating a role model, following in the footsteps of a mentor, or someone you admire; it's in the destructive mindset that sometimes accompanies those good intentions, which keeps you from realizing your own potential and discovering your own unique purpose.

So what did I do? First of all, I prayed for wisdom, and when I prayed for wisdom, I didn't yet realize everything I just shared with you. I was still under the impression that my way was 'working' and I didn't need any direction. But it wasn't. I was frustrated by my efforts that I began realizing were in vain. I became exhausted and it became difficult to stay motivated. But my prayer was answered and slowly the cloud lifted. I won't go into detail because I'm not writing this in order that you pray for wisdom so that all your struggles vanish, your path is laid out clearly in front of you, and all your worries and anxieties dissipate. I am, however, sharing this with you so that you understand that it's a process, and see that it's in this struggle; it's in this transition from Woman Number Two, to Woman Number One that you're being refined. Just like iron sharpens iron; diamonds are formed under great pressure; and pearls are created by the irritation of unpleasant circumstances, you can become your most beautiful self through trial and challenge

That said…

Everyone has days of insecurity. Everyone feels 'not good enough' at times. But that's a lie. That's a lie to keep you from realizing your true purpose. Want the truth? You were created by God, who loves you, and you have been uniquely gifted with certain talents, and insights, and wisdom, and a way to see the world that nobody else on the planet has, or ever has had, or ever will have because you are unique. As soon as you realize that, you'll be able to change the world.

Even if you can't see it now, even if you never see it yourself, you're here for a reason. I want you to know that beyond a shadow of a doubt. Own it. Believe it. Trust it. You are beautiful, unique, gifted, and nothing anybody says, or nothing you think will ever change that. The world needs your individuality. It also needs the positivity that comes from a woman who knows her value and understands the truth that she has something special that no one else can offer… herself.

You see, we all have unique talents and abilities, and dreams and goals, but what is the point of reaching those goals if only to reach them? The beauty lies not only in the accomplishment of a goal (because you realized your potential to get there), but in the process of sharing your gifts with others and inspiring them to do the same along the way; the secret isn't in discovering what you were meant to do, but in how you let God develop your character along the way. Ironically, that has nothing to do with personal betterment or 'self-improvement,' but it has everything to do with the encouraging, serving, and building up of others, especially those you may have seen as your competition before. Therein lies the irony. Because in building up, encouraging, blessing and loving others, you not only stop tearing your own house down, you start to rebuild it. And in the whole messy process, you become a better you.

Now, spend some time reflecting on this. Ask yourself, "which woman am I right now?" and "which woman am I becoming?". Then remember that there is only one you, and only one person who can do what you do the way you do it. Comparing yourself to others only reveals your own fear and insecurity, and will only delay you reaching your potential, and hurt others in the process. So instead, embrace your individuality, and shine, baby, shine!

"...As we let our own light shine, we unconsciously give other people permission to do the same. As we are liberated from our own fear, our presence automatically liberates others." - M. Williamson

Rachel Elizabeth Murray
I'm an LA based fitness spokes model and personality, model/actress, athlete, trainer/nutritionist and founder of CauseFitness.

The Awareness & Manifestation of Ego
by Karen Pang

Focus. Determination. Drive. These are just some of the characteristics associated with athletes who spend endless hours training, pushing, sweating and toiling over their sport all hours of the day. Their peers and fans elevate them to a pedestal of admiration with the motivation and inspirational achievements exuded through titles, trophies and magazine covers. There is also another trait that is ubiquitous and flows thoroughly in the veins of fitness/bodybuilding industry: Ego.

I will touch upon this subject with two different moods: formal analytical and idiomatic with a slight comedic twist.

Don't get me wrong; I'm not saying everyone in the fitness realm is a self absorbed, arrogant dumbbell-wielding narcissist. But coincidentally, bodybuilding has been regarded as a "selfish sport" and funny enough if you look up the definition of ego, its Latin word meaning "I" and is used in the English language relating to "self". The vast majority of us human beings possess ego, which is completely normal. The perfect ego in my opinion is a healthy ego, which falls between the blocks of high self-importance and low self-regard. Possessing humility, respect and integrity are just some of the traits of a healthy ego.

For those of you who have never competed or have had someone close to you compete, let me fill you in on a few things. Why bodybuilding is deemed a "selfish" sport is that the competitor's life is consumed training and diet. When they train, sleep, rise, what they eat, what they cannot eat, when they eat, why they won't too often engage in social events because of training or a restricted diet. It all revolves around them. There is no compromise. There is no room for error. This is part of the price they pay to win.

Let me begin with an example of a subject with a healthy ego who decides to compete in a physique competition. They win their show, people congratulate them, start to get attention from strangers and gets publicity through social media or magazines. These consecutive rewards are all great for their self-esteem, albeit based on superficial achievements. When the recognition and admiration starts to overflow, and one loses awareness and stability of the healthy ego it starts to slowly manifest itself. The attachment to the praise of others leads to belief and growing idealism that one is above their prior self and others and is ignorant to what is real and factual. This for example, is very common in the fitness scene. I've seen, heard and experienced it first hand.

I've met numerous people in the fitness industry. Some I loosely use the term "friends" and very few that I have close in my life. There have been people whom I've gotten to know and was so tired of one-sided conversations that I had distanced myself from them. From what I've gathered and taken inventory of, here are some telltale signs of an overactive ego. They:

- Refer to themselves in third person
- Introduce themselves with their first AND last name
- Give themselves nicknames
- Complain about people wanting to date/get to know them for who they are or how connected they are in the industry
- Are offended if you or anyone doesn't know who they are
- Are extremely nice to high profile industry people and could care less about others without titles

This goes with anyone, egomaniac or not that if anyone ever begins a sentence with "I am smart/humble/rich", it usually means they're not because if you're actually smart you would have a more subtle and intelligent way to say it. If you're humble, you wouldn't even say that in the first place and if you're rich and you say it...well, that means you're not smart so expect to get robbed.

Personally, even I have experienced a growing ego at one point. Everything was going right for me in the fitness scene, I was at my physical best, people were giving me compliments on how good I was looking so I was going into Nationals with confidence. Well, I got my butt handed to me on a silver platter. I was competing in figure at the time and was TINY compared to those other girls. A year later, I reverted to the category in which proved to be the most successful for me: Bikini. I thought it would be a piece of cake to win my IFBB Pro Card, but in my first year competing in the Canadian circuit I never claimed first place. I fell victim to other people's words: "You ARE bikini Karen", "You ARE a pro", "It's YOUR time". After seven Pro Qualifiers and three 1st place finishes, I gave up. I was over the mental anguish of not turning Pro, pushing my body and mind to exhaustion and truthfully, my ego had been bruised too many times. On a whim, I entered my last Nationals a week before the show and kept it low key. I didn't want to hear any well wishes, I just wanted to compete because I wanted to experience the original reason why I started: for the fun & love of competition and especially not for a Pro Card.

I haven't a romantic or philosophical way to bring anyone to the realization of the ego. All I request is that you experiment with yourself every once in a while beginning today, to treat a stranger as if they were you. Whether that person is a gas station attendant, waiter or someone asking for directions. Sometimes we're not very warm or welcoming because we judge people based on their appearance or status. But what makes us better than these people? Really? Do you do charitable work just for your ego or are you genuinely interested in making a difference in someone's life?

This topic has so many aspects that I can talk all day about, and the most difficult thing for me in this chapter in Miriam's book was to downsize and keep it concise. I really thank you for taking the time to read my chapter and I hope you enjoy the rest of this fabulous book!

Karen Pang

I'm a 3x Canadian national bikini champion, personal trainer & owner of KaBling Designs.

These 4 Words Could Change Your Life by Donna Richards and Tora Cullip

Donna looked right at that huge chunk of chocolate she was about to shove into her mouth and thought to herself, "Why am I doing this? Why am I breaking all the healthy habits that I've tried so hard to create for myself?" And, in that moment, she realized she felt too exhausted and fed up to care about her weight, her health or her wellbeing. It didn't matter, and she didn't matter.

Donna's work as an international facilitator and coach has meant she's spent many hours on the road - long-haul flights, strange hotels, irregular eating patterns and weird (not always wonderful!) cuisine. One year, only a few years back, she lost an entire month's worth of sleep due to her crazy, long haul travel schedule...and that doesn't include all the sleepless nights due to jetlag. Now that's a lot of sleep deprivation!

During a trip to Africa (a 30 hour flight from Australia), she was sitting in her hotel room one night and all she could think about was where her next caffeine or sugar hit was coming from. She was tired, homesick and didn't know how she'd summon up the energy for two more days of training people. Donna reached into her suitcase, brought out her emergency ration of chocolate and started to break off a huge chunk.

And that's when Donna realized something: with an "it doesn't matter, I don't matter" mindset, she was on the fast track to unhealthy food choices, skipping workouts, drinking too much (of anything but water), and self-sabotage.

This realization was quite a breakthrough. As a behavior change specialist, Donna is always on the lookout to help people understand how their behavior impacts their results, and what better way to learn than through her own experience? Donna knew that with a mindset that said "it doesn't matter", she would probably spend the next few days eating too much chocolate and other sugary snacks, drinking a lot of coffee and probably gaining a few pounds. Not ideal, but she also new that returning to her familiar routines could quickly restore the balance.

However, with an "I don't matter" mindset, she was really telling herself that she was unimportant, worthless and not good enough. Her inner dialogue was saying that it didn't matter what choices she made to take care of herself on another of her tiring trips overseas, because she didn't matter.

Most of us have a belief - anything from a quiet whisper to a loud roar - that tells us we're not good enough. If that belief is very strong there is little chance of being able to look, feel or be your best because there will always be a little voice that contradicts you, saying "but you don't matter.".

Donna and I believe that the "it doesn't matter, I don't matter" mindset lies at the heart of many weight, health and body confidence issues; it was certainly at the core of our own weight struggles. When I had an eating disorder, Anorexia Nervosa, my body weight plummeted to just 81lb and I could see every bone in my body. Even though I thought each pound lost would result in feeling better about my body, the reality is that as my weight dropped my self-loathing increased. I didn't think I mattered enough to love myself.

When Donna was 70lbs overweight, she thought so little of herself that it didn't matter what she ate, or how much of it, and she continued to yo-yo diet for over 7 years. Each time she tried to take charge of her weight or go on another diet, that little voice kicked in and she'd sabotage all of her success, ending up heavier than when she started.

Although Donna and I have come from opposite ends of the weight spectrum and have now been at our confident weight for over 15 years, our journeys to feeling comfortable in our own skin have been remarkably similar. We knew that our beliefs and thinking patterns had played havoc with our self-esteem and our weight came to represent just how little we loved and cared for ourselves. We both had to make changes to our mindset so that our weight stopped being the measuring stick for our worth.

Making the shift from a destructive mindset to "It Matters, I Matter" is one of the most powerful changes you can make to start loving yourself more. To help with this, we are both big believers in repeating affirmations to crowd out those negative, destructive belief patterns we have all held onto for so long.

Once Donna had identified the "It Matters, I Matter" mindset in her hotel room back in Africa, she started to practice this affirmation multiple times a day. Every time she reached for another cup of coffee, an afternoon cake or her emergency chocolate ration, she would say to herself: "It matters what I eat and drink, I matter.".

During those last few days of her trip, Donna started to make choices that made her feel good about how she was taking care of herself. Donna's the first to admit that she's no saint so she still enjoyed her morning coffee and some of her favorite chocolate, but she felt back in control. She was in the driver's seat of her weight, health and wellbeing - and it all came down to that simple, but powerful, shift in her mindset.

When we started to teach and coach people using this "It Matters, I Matter" mindset, we discovered that it had a profound impact for our clients too. They started to say "no" to the office donuts; cook more meals at home; have the courage to try a Zumba class for the first time; go to bed a little earlier; take time out for themselves. Most importantly, they felt a growing confidence in how they felt about themselves on the inside, which in turn made them want to look better on the outside.

If you want to start living more fully and loving yourself more, these four simple words could change your life: "It Matters, I Matter".

Go ahead, and start using them today!

Donna Richards & Tora Cullip

We are Body Confidence Specialists, on a mission to help women live at their confident weight through healthy habits, a joyful relationship with food and self-love, rather than fad diets, deprivation and self-loathing.

You Are Your Own 24/7
by Kristi Tauti

You are what you choose to be, your life will be a reflection of the choices you make in response to what the world gives you. I have always been a person that will look at each situation and figure out how I need to climb each mountain/hurdle in life, rather than, why way I given this mountain or using the mountain as an excuse to quit.

I grew up in a small town of about 1,500 people and learned quickly to make things happen for me, rather than wait for them to be handed to me. Simply put, I love HARD WORK and I thrive off of accomplishing goals. A quote I feel reflects my life is "Respect is earned when no one is looking." This is where the hard work is applied in building the foundation of your goals and persevering until it is accomplished.

About 2 years ago I began quite a new journey that required extreme perseverance. My husband and I opened our own iPhysique Gym which was a big goal, but we had very minimal business experience. Exactly 2 months after we opened our gym, I gave birth to my 2nd child. This was a challenge as I was the prime revenue source for the gym but could only work minimally for the first month of my sons life. While struggling with the balance of business owner and new motherhood, I also had to be the Coach and Leader to a team of 35 active Bodybuilding/Figure/Bikini competitors. I coached them to show while, running the gym, running my family, and beginning my own contest prep. I am an IFBB Professional Figure athlete and have been competing for 12 years but my contest prep this time was very challenging with what I had on my plate of responsibilities. I was successful and was able to step on stage 6.5 months after giving birth to my son, Levai.

I have an 8 year old daughter Talia that has such a tender heart and is always supportive of my goals, but it is important to me that I do not bring the struggles of my competition prep into our home. She would not know whether I am in prep or not unless I tell her. It is also important to me that she see's me as a positive role model who loves to be active and who has a passion for clean eating. I know that I am planting the seeds that will allow her to make the choices in her life that will keep her healthy and happy.

I have recently taken a passion to outdoor obstacle racing and other athletic or performance based events as opposed to the physique based events I have done for the last 12 years. This new passion has allowed me to keep Talia more involved and active with me in a way that she can enjoy. We can go to the playground and I will train on the monkey bars, jump rope, balance beam, climbing the pole etc. What better way can a child stay active then to enjoy it with her mother. I feel very balanced being able to incorporate my family life with my fitness life and not let the fitness become a negative thing that takes my time away from my children.

We have also discovered that the best way to incorporate clean eating is to get the kids in the grocery store and kitchen with you. Yes it will take more time than if you were to do it on your own, but it is quality time that teaches invaluable lessons to my child.

Here are some tips that we have enjoyed:

Going through the grocery store and using the "fooducate" phone app to scan foods that have a label and grades them. She cannot purchase something that is lower than a C+. Along with that she has to choose as many whole foods as she can.

Talia started her own garden in our backyard that she calls "her business" because she is feeding our family. She enjoys watering her plants and talks to them to help them grow.

When we have smaller grocery trips Talia enjoys using the self scan to scan our purchases and bag them, she organizes the categories of fruits, vegetables etc.

In the kitchen cutting the fruits and veggies is even more exciting to her now that she gets to use an adult knife. (Under adult supervision of course!)

Making videos of her in the kitchen making clean eating recipes (she doesn't eat most of them yet but enjoys making them for me). Kids love to see themselves on video and even more if you post it on Facebook and they see your friends' comments.

I train clients, competitors and athletes of all levels and find that those who are most successful are those that follow my advice and learn to "live in the grey." I say that meaning that if you make a mistake you acknowledge and correct as soon as possible.

Those that dwell in their mistake, or expect nothing but perfection, will find themselves running around in circles and never getting anywhere, or frustrating themselves to the point that they feel defeated. Along with that I strongly believe that "You are your own 24/7" you must take personal responsibility for your actions rather than putting the blame on others. Too many times we fail to be true to ourselves and no one else knows exactly what you do in the 24 hours that are given to you daily. If I am in the house alone (which is rare) I do not go to the cupboard to sabotage my diet or clean eating lifestyle because I would not be true to myself and would only be hurting.

My hope is that I have inspired you find ways or reasons to succeed in life, rather than finding excuses as to why you did not succeed.

Have a happy and healthy life, be inspiring, and bring balance to life.

Real Talk Real Women

Kristi Tauti

I'm an IFBB figure pro athlete, nutritionist, entrepreneur and coach. I'm also the proud mom of 2, a GNC sponsored athlete and the owner / operator of iPhysiqueGym.

The Tale of "The Barbell Pickup" by Erica Willick

A metal bar with two round weighted circles holds more power than meets the eye. To my friend Karen she saw in that innate piece of gym equipment an intimidating reminder of what she couldn't yet do on her own in her life. Karen is a successful woman by anyone's standards. She has a career, two children, a loving marriage, and had already lost 40lbs as part of a mom weight loss group.

Each program Karen was given by a trainer used dumbbells not the barbell, and so she continued to dubiously eye up her opponent at the gym.

At 5 a.m. one morning, I sat on the edge of a weight bench in the gym ready to lean back into my barbell chest press and I thought of Karen. Years had passed since I felt like the gym was anything other than my second home, a safe haven, and a spot for sweat therapy. But that morning I remembered my former self, a woman who was new to the weight room, unsure of her surroundings and most significantly unsure of herself. I leaned all the way back on the bench, positioned myself under the loaded barbell, grasped the metal bar with my gloved hands, breathed in, and pushed. I pushed for me and I pushed for Karen.

I told Karen I had picked up the barbell in her honour that morning and expected her to join me soon. Karen promised she was getting her nerve up and soon would venture out to the co-ed weight room to go toe-to-toe with the barbell.

A couple weeks passed and Karen wrote: "Well I did it – I picked up the barbell for my squats today! Wow! I loved it. I was able to squat deeper than I ever have and really felt it in my legs...I felt like superwoman!!"

And then the next week Karen wrote "I did my entire program on the 'boys' side of the gym today! I used equipment I've never used before. I'm feeling good after stepping way out of my comfort zone. Baby-steps but I'm making progress."

And then the next week Karen wrote "I feel so empowered, I taught myself how to use the smith machine today and was able to add more plates! I became less and less self-conscious as the workout went on. I'm feeling so good. This is just the beginning for me."

And then Karen wrote what I know is really the game-changer when it comes to lasting health & fitness:

"If I can keep this powerful feeling going, then I know anything is possible and my dreams will happen!"

I grinned from ear to ear, and felt my own sense of empowerment start to vibrate. The barbell was the same as it was before, but with a single shift of perspective Karen grabbed a hold of her power and was different. Karen was empowered.

Recently Karen beautifully shared "I have always been self-conscious of my legs. I've always thought of them as thick and big. Last week I took a huge step out of my comfort zone and bought the shortest workout shorts I've ever bought in my life and today I actually wore them! For the first time I looked in the mirror and loved the athletic legs I saw. I can see my hard work paying off and I wasn't self-conscious at all. It may seem silly but for me wearing short workout shorts in public is a giant leap for me!"

Karen shows how each small action builds, just like moments build time into years and years into decades. Yet we often feel the answers in our own health and fitness are beyond our own knowledge and abilities. That somehow exercise and food has become so complicated it is best left to the direction by experts. So we give up our power.

But who is the expert on your health? Your doctor? The nutritionist that has 10 accreditations behind his name? What about that lady who writes all those books? She must know what you should do. And really who are you to know more than they do? You're just a busy average woman who maybe has a kid or two (or three), so it's probably best to let the experts point you in the right direction.

You see Karen grasped what is the key to lasting health the day she chose to allow her fear and uncertainty to keep her company while she picked up that barbell. Empowerment. The power to choose and the power to act.

Erica Willick
I'm an accountant mommy bikini champ.

VOLUME II - NEVER GIVE UP

Fitness Saved Our Lives; Two Sister's Journey by Elizabeth Aguilera & Morgan Wehmer

Elizabeth's Journey

My name is Elizabeth Aguilera and I am a cancer survivor, military spouse and recent Purdue graduate. My sister and I have two powerful fitness journeys. In a three-year time span I have survived cancer while simultaneously dealing with military deployments, 4 cross country moves with the military, graduating top ten percent from Purdue and placing fourth place in my first NPC competition. Looking back on those three years, I can honestly say they were the hardest times of my life and because of them I am not the woman I used to be. Through fighting the disease and cancer we have strived even harder to not only overcome our illnesses, but reach new goals we have always thought were out of reach. We are now motivational speakers, certified personal trainers, Oh Yeah! Athletes and Lifestyle Leaders, NPC competitors, and published fitness models with Naturally Fit.

I used fitness as an outlet to transform my life and create a stronger mind and body to help me reach my goals. My sister, Morgan, has a powerful story as well. Through overcoming anorexia and deciding to regain her health through proper nutrition and workout regimen she has changed her life completely. Living a healthy lifestyle has transformed our bodies and minds. We chose to be fighters and never give up hope.

We are not your typical cookie cutter success story. Most of the media portray motivating stories focused upon men and women's weight loss journeys. We chose to share our two experiences to shed light on the fact that there are people everyday who are battling cancer and disease but in this industry it's hard for people to talk about these topics. After all, it is not an easy topic to speak of. We want to show people going through disease and illness that just like us they too can change their lives. We are here to show you that fitness is not only about weight loss. A healthy lifestyle is not just about physical health and having a "hot body." It is about maintaining a balance with physical, mental and spiritual health.

Essentially, it is the hardest times that will shape you into the stronger person who you have always wanted to be. The road to success is full of challenges. Always. You have to be fearless. Wake up every morning and challenge yourself to fight. Be a better version of yourself everyday. When was the last time you tried something new? Everyday, every morning, give yourself the opportunity to fight for what you want and step into the unknown territory. It is going to be uncomfortable to fight when you are stressed, scared, feel alone or want to give up but that is when the magic is going to happen. The painful times molded our weaknesses into newfound strength and taught us how to live and cherish our health, and how to take pride in our bodies and minds.

We all have battles each and everyday that is forced into our presence. While trying to deal with these battles some of us revert to bad habits, which can often lead to a downward spiral. Mental will is like a muscle. When you practice being strong, it becomes a new habit. Think about it. Eventually how you live one day will end up how you live your life. By changing small habits each day we can transform our lives completely. It is inevitable that change and stress will enter our lives at some point or another. After all, you can't spell challenge without "change." Accept that life is full of change. Accept that you can't plan your life. Accept the choice to be a fighter and take the hits as they come. The only aspect you are in control of is your attitude. Accept that and from there you will find peace.

By sharing our stories we want to inspire people. We want someone to look at us and say, "because of you, I did not and will not give up".

Think about how you take out the trash everyday in your home. Could you image how it would be with over a month or year of trash if you chose to not take it all out? Now vision your mind. It is no different. Take out the trash and reach for mental clarity. Know that even if you have painful experiences or trials standing in your way that you will throw away those thoughts of fear and stress and use that energy to create positive changes. That is how I have gotten through my military stresses with my husband and still to this day how I deal with my cancer.

My journey began at age 20 when I married my husband who enlisted in the US Navy. I began online classes at Purdue and moved to begin my husband's career. During the next 3 years, I moved cross-country a total of 4 times! During this time I was doing endless cardio and eating low calories. I was not finding the results I wanted and I decided to invest in a nutritionist. From there I went 24% body fat to 12% eating 5-6 healthy meals a day and learning the importance of nutrition. My husband then left for his first deployment, and I felt I had reached my nutrition and fitness goals.

I felt that I had really gained control of my life. I had learned the correct way to eat and workout and was doing exceptionally well in my classes while my husband returned from the Middle East. It was too good to be true it seemed, as my advisor informed me that I had to return to Purdue for my last year of classes since the online classes were running out. I decided to move back home to finish my last year of college. I thought this was the last hard step my husband and I would have to overcome. We just went through multiple cross-country moves and we had gotten through his deployment, so we thought after graduation everything would start to become smooth sailing!

The week before I was planning on moving home, I went to the doctor to get my yearly physical. My insured doctors must be military based, so since I wouldn't have them back at home and I thought it was important that I get a check up before leaving. That is where I found out I had melanoma. Since that August of 2012, I had 4 surgeries and 7 areas removed.

I moved home and began the classes like a normal student. My professors and even my mother told me the best thing to do would be to drop the classes since I was flying to Florida to see my doctors every 3 weeks.

I didn't drop a single class. It was very stressful, time consuming and draining. I remember sitting in my kitchen after I got off the phone with my doctor and I was so mad at my life and at God. I looked back and saw the past years of obstacles I'd had thrown my way and I just asked, "why can't I ever have a break?"

I couldn't relate to my friends or anyone who had these types of problems and felt it was unfair. I really hit a low point in my life. On top of the cancer I was also told my husband would be sent for another deployment after I graduated in May. So the whole time I was home at school and having to go to all these surgeons and doctors left me no time to really be with him and then he was leaving for another 6 months? It was a lot to take in.

I was at my lowest and I decided that all I could do was pray. I prayed to just be a stronger person to get through this and I put my life in his hands. I felt everything was so out of control that the only thing I could do was my best. I went from trying to control every aspect of my life to understanding that life can and will throw anything my way.

I never knew what was coming next but I did know that I was going to handle it the best way I could. In the end I knew my trials were going to shape every detail of me.

Resisting the inevitable, complaining and feeling sorry for myself did absolutely nothing, so I decided to simply change my attitude. Presently, my husband just left for his deployment and my melanoma will be with me forever, but I have accepted it and how things are.

Now, every two months I go to the doctor for my exams, which consist of full body screenings, lymph node exams and cat scans to monitor everything. This past September of 2013 I will also be having another melanoma area removed for the second time. This illness will be something I have to live with everyday and watch carefully, but with maintaining a positive attitude I will get through it.

Life is too short! I really feel that my apparent obstacles are actually blessings in disguise and they have made me appreciate my loved ones, my life, and really focus on my health.

You are capable of anything you put your mind to. Whether you think you can or you think you can't, you are RIGHT.

Morgan's Journey

My personal fitness journey was a mental challenge as well as a psychological and physical challenge. This is never an easy topic to discuss but the relevancy of such an issue is unbelievable as many men and women suffer from related issues but are too fearful to seek help. Let alone make vast and crucial changes. I had battled a severe eating disorder throughout my entire high school career. At the time, my life seemed completely out of my own control. I was suffering from the stresses of failing relationships and a very difficult family life. I felt that I, myself, had no control of my own life or the events taking place in it. In my mind, the only thing I felt that I could control, however, was every morsel I put into my mouth. I soon began to react to my problems by controlling every bite I took, causing me to lose over 30 pounds. Looking at me now, I stands at 145 pounds. So if you can imagine me at about 115 pounds, you may be able to picture the severity.

I went through a few years where family and friends tried to reach out and help me in what ways they knew how, but finally I decided to 'retrain my brain' and create a short term goal then more short term goals and so on. These goals varied from calorie goals that I wanted to hit for the day, positive affirmations, and even researching a new nutrition or exercise facts or physiological information that would help myself work to become better and stronger than the average person going about their healthy lifestyle. I wanted to not only put this disease in my past, but through it, to become better, healthier and more fit than I ever thought possible.. And I did.

I now have more willpower than one can imagine, more concern for others who are in such situations, and most importantly I now care and value my body as the temple it truly is. I have been able to reach out to so many women who have experienced similar fights and I make my absolute best effort to spread my knowledge and power of will to any neighbor in need of it. I can safely state that I would not be where I am today, helping, inspiring, teaching, and cherishing my body and health.. WITHOUT having overcome such a disease. These is yet another example of how you must take your past and use it to better your future. And do this with no regrets.

I feel that it is of utmost importance to address this issue as you are probably encountering people with like struggles more often than you may think. This is something that the average person does not want to make known to the public eye. This also is definitely not something one intrinsically knows how to fix or may even be at the stage where anyone's help is welcomed.

Because of that, it is important to understand the relevancy of this issue and that there absolutely IS a way to surpass it, just as there is a way to surpass anything you set your mind to.

Since this battle, I have gained over 30 pounds of muscle to my frame. I have a stronger body and mind, and am lucky enough to be able to help others see that they can, indeed, achieve just that as well. My passion for health has also inspired me to apply for the IU nursing program where I was one of the 60 students accepted out of over 1000 applicants to the program. My determination and passion for health has forever changed my life. And fortunately I have now even been able to change others' lives through this.

We have also created our own website and social media sites to motivate and encourage others to live a healthy lifestyle. On our sites we post daily workouts, nutrition tips, motivational posts and recipes. Everyday we motivate our followers to never give up and to fight for their goals. What seem to be bitter trials are often blessings in disguise. We are happy when God answered our prayers but we are more thankful when God is letting us answer to someone else's prayers.

Elizabeth Aguilera & Morgan Wehmer
We are Oh Yeah! Nutrition Lifestyle Leaders, NPC competitors, published fitness models, motivational speakers, writers and certified trainers.

The Three C's of Fitness Success
by Christine Anderson

COMMITMENT, CONSISTENCY, and a CAN-DO ATTITUDE are important in achieving and maintaining your fitness goals. When you combine these three qualities with achievable goals, you will begin to see the fruits of your labor in your fitness journey. Many times I see a client's fitness journey begin to positively influence other areas of their life: better time management and built up confidence levels which then permeates into their careers and relationships. I'm not trying to be negative but the opposite holds true, too. If you fail to be committed, consistent, and apply a can-do attitude to your fitness goals, your frustration will be felt in the day-to-day things of your life!

A personal COMMITMENT to your fitness success must be paramount in your life. As a mother, putting the needs of our children comes first and we would go to great lengths to protect them. I'm not saying your fitness goals should come before your children, what I am saying is being healthier and feeling better does require you to place your needs high on the list. I'm a firm believer that a healthy mom is a happy mom. No one else will do it for you so YOU must make that decision and stick with it no matter what. When I perform a consultation, I will ask on a scale of 1 to 10, what is their commitment level to their training and nutrition program, 1 being not committed and 10 being very committed? Personal trainers are a great source to push, motivate, and hold you accountable but having a commitment level that is less than 8 may become a struggle for you and a waste of money. If hiring a Personal Trainer is not possible at the time, telling a close friend of your fitness goal puts the accountability out there and will cause you to think twice before ordering fries with your shake. Commitment starts with a simple, realistic goal. If your goal is to lose 50lbs and you decide you want to lose that in 2 months, this is not only unrealistic but becomes discouraging if not lost within the time frame you set. It's probably a better idea to break up the 50lb into a smaller number, say 15lbs in 2 months where the goal is achievable. Losing 1-2lbs per week may not sound exciting but it is an achievable and healthier approach versus a quick weight loss, which is normally due to a fad diet or severe calorie restriction. In order to attain your long-term vision, you must be able to conquer your short-term vision and before you know it, you will compete in your very first fitness competition!

CONSISTENCY in your fitness program can lead to a lifestyle change that will help you to keep the results you worked so hard for. Every person I know that is on their way to achieving their fitness goal will have setbacks. This is part of the process and completely normal, and when this happens get back on track and keep moving forward. Have more good days than bad days and the outcome will always get you to your goal. Before I had my daughter, Nohea, I was schedule driven (some things never change even after she was born). Then when I gave birth to her, with her eating schedule and my eating schedule, I became a schedule-holic! I found myself eating every 3 hours, she's eating every 2 hours, and this eating business became a full time job between the two of us! The consistency of properly fueling the body gave me the energy needed to be efficient and get great workouts. Not only are you feeling better at home, work, or school, your energy- fueled workouts are helping your body burn calories. Time management becomes your best friend because you are making healthy eating and workouts part of your life. Most health experts say it takes 21 days to break a habit. So while you are diligently working to break an old habit, you are also in the process of developing new healthy habits. Some basic consistencies you can begin with are to eat 4-5 meals a day and spread them every 2-3 hours. Time your workout meals so you eat 45 minutes – 1 hour before a workout and within 30 minutes post workout. If your body is properly fueled and hydrated for your pre and post workout, you created a fat burning window for the body.

When starting a fitness journey, it starts off as a physical feat but the longer you are on this journey it becomes more of a mental challenge to push through the really tough moments. Approach every fitness goal with a CAN-DO ATTITUDE!

You know you need to be committed and consistent, but sometimes we can be our worst enemy in our mind. We place everyone else's needs in front of ours but we need to be stronger than that and DO IT. I call it, 'mentally checking in' or 'get your head in the game'.

Your work, school, and home environment can positively or negatively affect the way you think and feel. Choose to be around those that will support you and your new lifestyle. If you don't have a support system, stay focused on your goal and as you start getting results these non-supporters will either leave you alone or become fans.

Set a short and long term goal for yourself, next set a vision of what you want to look like. I'm a visual person and like to have an idea of what I want to look like. It motivates me to work towards what I think is an ideal image in my head.

You know, like sticking a fitness model's photo on the fridge to deter you from opening it to search for something you aren't supposed to eat? All of us have an idea of what we would like to look like, before you know it you created your own fitness image and you are now a successful before and after story.

Miriam Khalladi

Christine Anderson

I'm a personal trainer, fitness coach, business owner, busy wife and mother to one extraordinary girl!

Fear of Failure
by Robyn Baldwin

We are not born with the fear of failure. As we grow and learn to walk we have the belief that we will get up and walk. We are all born as optimists. And when we attempt those first steps to walk, we have supportive parents cheering us on. They are there holding out their hands to catch us if we fall. If we stumble, we get right back up and keep trying. We are determined and nothing can stop us.

What happened along the way to give us trepidation, hesitation and that scared feeling? As we grow older we experience failures and setbacks. We learn an emotional reaction to these acts of "failure" which, we try to avoid as we grow older and move through life, so that we don't have to go through these emotions again.

The emotional reaction can be described as the feeling that your heart is sinking into your chest, or that an imaginary hand is gripping your heart so tightly that you can't breathe, can't think and have no idea what to do.

What personal "failures" have I experienced? I have been let go from a job; I've broken up with long-term boyfriends; I've had to cancel a wedding to a man I thought I'd spend the rest of my life with; I've competed in fitness competitions and not placed; I've gone after running certain time race goals and not achieved them. What I want to say here is that "failure" can come in so many different moments in life. Failures are personal due to your expectations. They don't have to be "big" in terms of society to elicit an upsetting emotional reaction.

Any event that happens in your life where you feel like you haven't lived up to a certain expectation, either set by yourself or those around you, can be seen as a failure. The moment or event of failure could be something you could have controlled or maybe you had no control over the situation. A failure is not easily defined, but it can be felt in so many different ways.

By telling you about different failures in my life I want to explain that they can come in so many different ways throughout life. They can come from goals I've set for myself or from life events that were supposed to happen. Failure has not always been ever so present in my life. When I first experienced a "major" failure of being let go from a job, I thought it was embarrassing. How can a self-proclaimed Alpha Female fail at anything in life? And then I stopped thinking that way, because I acknowledged that I'm human and imperfect. Anything and everything that I've gone through in my life makes me, me. In moments of failure I would wonder why it was happening. But on the other side of failure I can now say I'm grateful for every single experience. I'm grateful for the journey no matter how difficult it has been.

I'm sure I'm going to fail at things again in the future. It's inevitable, but from my broken-heel moments so far I now know steps to take to get me back on track. Here are 10 things you can slowly incorporate into your life when you're ready, and in no particular order, to help you heal and get back on your life path.

1. **Feel Your Feelings**

You are allowed to feel whatever way you feel. Allow yourself to feel. Then allow yourself to work through those feelings. Ask yourself: Why do you feel that way? How can you move through it, past it? I completely recommend going to see a psychiatrist or psychotherapist or therapist or whatever floats your boat. I went to see a cognitive therapist after calling off my wedding to work through everything that was going on in my head. I asked in my first session what the purpose of therapy was as I was never a believer that it was something I was ever going to need in life.

My therapist told me that, hopefully at the end of each session, I would feel a little bit lighter. I would never have all the answers, but I would feel lighter. And that feeling of being slightly lighter each time helped me heal and take it one day at a time.

2. **Grieve**

I didn't want to cry. I didn't want to feel hurt. I didn't want to feel weak. I kept getting so mad at myself for crying. I have come to realize that until you release an emotion it will tie you down. It will make you drag your feet on the ground. So grieve. It's hard to write instructions on how to grieve. If I can offer any advice it would be to just let the hurt happen and then let it go. I also can't define what "let it go" will mean for you. It could be forgiveness; it could be refocusing on a new goal. It is different in every moment of failure and unique to individuals. Grief is a process and is different for everyone, but in my moments of failure I didn't want to acknowledge sad feelings. I wanted to be "stronger" than them. But I am human. I feel, oh boy do I cry, and that is ok.

3. **Read Quotes**

When I first discovered Pinterest I found boundless fashion ideas, wedding visions and quotes. The first three boards I created were for Fitness Inspiration, My Dream Wedding (as I was planning mine from January 2011 to July 2012) and my Words of Motivation quote board. Little did I know that in September 2012 I'd be turning to the platform to find solace in words? When insomnia hit, or emotions welled up too much or I was paralyzed in bed unable to move I kept my mind busy by playing iPhone games (so much that I overdosed on bejeweled) and by slowly scrolling through quote after quote on Pinterest. I sought solace in quotes that could explain my circumstances and gave me hope for the future. My Words of Motivation board has been added to over and over again and you can even see a theme of hurt to healing in the quotes that I've pinned over the past year. I have become addicted to quotes. I'm ok with this addiction. It's similar to my fitness addiction. If it benefits your life, it's a healthy obsession. I've also discovered that sharing quotes on my social networks is helping me connect with others who need words to heal. I'm grateful for those connections.

4. Surround Yourself with Positive People

Lean on your support system. I was lucky to have girlfriends, my mom, my dad & brother, co workers, acquaintances and social media friends swoop in with kind words, hugs and whatever was needed at the time. I leaned on them and I will be forever grateful for help getting over hurdles. Hugs heal. Sitting talking with a great listener heals. Watching chick flicks and eating ice cream or having tea / coffee dates heals. Going to beautiful yoga studios and being present on your mat beside your girls heals. Sometimes you just need to be with your support system and have them present in your life to heal.

5. Beware of the Curious

Our society loves drama. We crave it. We've been conditioned through reality TV, celebrity stalking and how open social media is. Beware in the midst of failure that there will be those who are offering to be part of your support system but are generally just in it for the curiosity. Be careful of who you open up to, as it can hinder the healing process later if trust is broken.

6. Find Your Happy

I am not being paid in any way by this author but go and buy The

Happiness Project. If you have not read it yet do it now and take what you need from the book to build your own project. If you've read it but haven't had a chance to start your own project yet, same thing goes for you. Do it now. Thank me later!

7. Make Bucket Lists

Wake up and live. Choose to live your life the way you want to and do things that make you happy. So choose your happiness project and start setting short-term and long-term goals. Dream and make yourself a bucket list of what you want to achieve over coming weeks or months.

8. Fitness Routine

There were days when my couch wouldn't let me off of it. It was so warm and comforting. However, on the days I forced myself to go to the gym and forced myself to sweat were good days. When a workout produces happy hormones (endorphins) that rush through your blood, it's just a little bit more possible to see the light at the end of the tunnel.

9. Eat Clean

Eat that bucket of ice cream. Order that extra large pizza all to yourself. Do it once and then stop. Emotionally eating is a slippery slope. I gained unhealthy weight when I ate emotionally to get through moments. I know now that I needed something comforting, but I also know that there comes a moment when you stop and say what really matters is good clean and healthy food to make me feel better. I spent time on meal plans and grocery shopping instead of feeling sorry for myself. I chose to fuel and nourish my soul. So getting back into a fitness routine and eating properly the way I had been before was exactly what I needed to give myself a foundation for healing.

10. Sleep

If you can sleep, sleep. Try and get those coveted 8 hours. Your body needs to heal from the stress it's going through and getting that great night sleep will lower your stress hormone cortisol. If you have insomnia then see your doctor for what you may need but I was able to use just melatonin or 5HTP and discussing dosage with my naturopath. I had to stop using the melatonin because I would have such vivid dreams that weren't always the most pleasant.

In Tosca Reno's words that she shared when speaking at the Can Fit Pro Conference in August 2103: we are all resilient human beings who can float.

I urge you to float.

Robyn Baldwin
I'm a self-branded Alpha Female. A former CFL cheerleader now published fitness model and writer, a fitness competitor, author, FitFluential ambassador, Magnum athlete and marketing manager at Kobo.

Overcoming Obstacles to Achieve Your Goals & Dreams
by Amy Bella

What haven't you done for a long time that brings you joy or a sense of achievement? Life is full of all the things we need to do and have to do, which is what life brings. We seem to think our dreams dry up when we become adults, parents or professionals. Involving yourself in activities that you enjoy but haven't found the time to do for years can help to bring a sense of life back to you and put you on the path to success, in any area you might find yourself in. It can lift your spirits, which will in turn make you feel as though you can do anything you set your mind to achieve.

Make a list and see if there's something that's keeping you from feeling free and alive. Are irrational thought processes holding you back? Unspoken words, unfinished projects, conversations, or skeletons in our closets can draw us away from what's important.

Share your goals & dreams! Most of us do not take this step because if we tell someone they might expect us to do something about it. Our instincts are to avoid the unfamiliar. Taking a chance and reaching out to someone means sharing our dreams with others, which makes us more accountable for achieving our dreams. When we have this healthy pressure to succeed we are more likely to work diligently to achieve our dreams and goals.

Schedule time; Take some time to write. Don't worry about your dream's possibilities or limitations… Just let go and write about what you truly want. Visualizing your dreams is imperative to achieving them. It is very difficult to achieve a dream if you are not able to visualize yourself enjoying the sweet victory of success.

Follow your heart and act on something that you know to be true for you. Show yourself that you are committed to at least exploring your dreams and prove to yourself that it's important by doing something. With anything that's consists of change or something that is important to us, living to reach your full potential includes being authentic and compassionate. Trade the ordinary for the extraordinary. Each day that is given to us is precious and unique from the previous day and from what will come tomorrow. In the end, you can say, "I truly lived my life, I gave it my all."

Wherever there is an obstacle, simply create a plan to drive around it or right through it. We often make obstacles larger than they are which can lead to the failure of our dreams. Identify what's stopping you from asking friends for help. Then be determined and dedicated in following through.

By taking these steps, you can achieve your goals and dreams.

Be inspiring to everyone around you! Show up ready, determined and outrageous. Let your creative spirit and beautiful bright light shine. Be the spark that ignites passion at home, at work and for other people you encounter. Show everyone what it means to be a true dreamer, by following your heart and encouraging others to do the same.

Inspiring others to achieve can give you the confidence that you need to achieve your own goals and dreams. To inspire means, "to breathe." And as oxygen is necessary for life, so inspiration is to dreaming. Discover what moves you. Dance, sing or simply express the feeling of the moment.

Live the fullest and most exciting adventure of life! Fear and excitement feel the same way for most of us. Push through these moments of adrenalin-fueled doubt. Keep going when your palms are sweating and your heart is pounding. Assume you have more capabilities than you know, then give it all you've got.

When you truly challenge yourself, you often find that you are capable of achieving more than you have ever dreamed of! It is through these times that we truly find out what we are made of.

In order to move your dream forward you must recognize and accept your past failures and disappointments. Use them as fuel to create the inferno inside as a driving force to guide you on the right path to success!

Create a project you can succeed within one month or less. Accomplishing small goals will help you build the confidence that you need to achieve bigger goals and dreams. Think about the outcomes you want, not all the details and make sure this goal is attainable. Track your progress along the way. Don't forget to celebrate when have reached your goals. Recognizing your success will inspire you to succeed even more. Take things one step at a time so you can achieve all your goals and dreams!

Never try and duplicate or emulate someone that is already successful in the hopes you too, will have their results. Be yourself, find your purpose, your talents, and share them with the world, and by doing this, you will become the inspiring force that motivates those around you.

Be you. Be a Champion!

By taking some of these steps, you can find ways to achieve your goals and dreams.

"I never said it would be easy, but I know it is worth it."

Amy Bella

I'm a 33 year old mother of 5 beautiful children with an amazing husband that helps support and guide me along this amazing journey we call life!

Unbreakable
by Carla Maria Cadotte

I don't really know where to begin with my story but I'll start with a brief introduction about myself I suppose. My name is Carla Maria Cadotte and I am a 31 year old Personal Trainer and Nutritional Consultant, model, and Fitness Competitor currently residing in Los Angeles, CA. I am a college graduate with my Bachelor's in Business Administration and Marketing from California State University of Fullerton, though I am originally from the San Francisco Bay Area.

I am a Childhood Sexual Abuse Survivor, Rape Survivor, and Domestic Violence Survivor, and a recovering addict with 4 years clean and sober, an ex stripper, I am proud of who I am today, but above all else, I am UNBREAKABLE.

Since I am not much of a writer, I will just begin with my personal story and journey that has made me the woman I am today. Looking at me most people would never guess the trials and tribulations I have endured throughout my life. Oftentimes people look at me, and based on my outward appearance, demeanor, and dress, they assume that I am a privileged woman whose beauty has provided her with an easier than normal life, or that I am lacking in intelligence, grew up with money, you name it I've heard it all.

However, very few aside from those who know me personally know that I am about as real of a person as it gets and that in the 31 years I have been alive, I have faced challenges that would break down most permanently.

With 4 years clean and sober, I am a recovering addict from prescription pills and cocaine, addictions that nearly destroyed my physical body, and my entire life from the time I was 16 years old until and 26 years old. But more important than the story of my past addiction is the story of what had taken me to such a point to begin with.

I grew up in an upper middle class suburb with loving parents, a tightly knit Filipino family, and an exceptional education. Most people would assume from initial glance that my life was "perfect" or that I had an "ideal upbringing." My childhood in its earliest years was one full of love and joy, and I was surrounded by family and friends at all times.

However, around the age of 8 years old, during the time that my father was completing his Residency for Medical School, I became the victim of Childhood Sexual Abuse and Incest by one of my uncles, and later in time another relative; a nightmare that would continue on a regular basis for about 6 more years of my life, a nightmare that would eventually lead me to years of depression, emotional pain and suffering, drug abuse, verbally and physically abusive relationships, love relationship issues, and hardship before leading me to my passion and life's purpose.

The sexual abuse I endured as a child was terribly painful and isolating for me, I still remember the feelings of sadness, loneliness, anxiety, depression, shame, hopelessness, confusion, anger, and fear that I felt everyday and for years to come.

Like many other sexual abuse survivors, I did not have a normal childhood. I grew up with a fear that "all men wanted to do things to me sexually" and a deep inner sadness stemming from the confusion and anger surrounding my abuse.

By the time I was 13 years old though I was still a Straight A student and a varsity athlete, I had begun drinking alcohol regularly, abusing prescription drugs, and experimenting heavily with illicit drugs as a means to escape the pain of the secrets I carried inside. By the time I was 15 years old my grades had started to fall and my behavior had become so bad that my mother began to try and figure out what was fueling my defiance. It was around this time that my mother went through my diaries and read my entries in which I had written about my abuse, thus uncovering my secret.

I was ridiculed and made fun of by peers when my abuse was discovered, and disbelieved by members of my own family when diaries I had written about my abuse in were read. Perhaps the most painful aspect of my sexual abuse was the lack of support I received from my family and most of my friends once the truth had come out, where rather than believing me and helping me to get the "help" I truly needed, I was told to basically pretend as if nothing had happened and that it would be "dealt with," by sending me off to a psychiatrist, and doped up on antidepressants without the type of counseling I truly needed to recover. When my secrets were revealed I remember being so relieved at first, but when I was met with questioning and blame by my family, the shame I already carried inside of me worsened, causing me to dive deeply into drug addiction by the time I was 18 years old.

By the age of 17 I was such a misfit that my father was threatening to kick me out of our home on a regular basis. Sadly, he had no idea about what had happened to me and thought I was simply being a rebellious teenager. The arguing at home was so horrible between my father and I that I moved out a few months before my 18th birthday.

When I was 18 years old, while I was completing my high school diploma at a local community college, I decided to take on a job as a stripper in San Francisco to help me support myself. Choosing such a profession was a personal choice I made for myself, a decision of which I have no regrets for as it served its purpose for the time being, and in my opinion a profession that is often misunderstood and I have a great deal of respect for the women in the business who are utilizing it as a means to an end.

Becoming a stripper, which I was for about 8 years of my adult life, was something that I did out of desperation as a young girl trying to survive, but was a job I was able to emotionally handle due to the lack of connection I felt to my physical body as a result of having my body abused and used for so many years at such a young age.

Although I do not believe in having regrets as I am proud of who I am and embrace all my faults and life experiences good and bad, the craziness of such a lifestyle and the abuse that one will endure working in it is oftentimes horrifying and was a huge factor in the worsening of my drug addiction.

In addition, during my time working as a stripper I worked in cities including San Francisco, Los Angeles, Hawaii, Las Vegas, and New Orleans, and a very prevalent trend was that in my experience about 90% of the women I met in the industry were also childhood sexual abuse survivors as well. Though I am not a psychologist I have always believed that the reason so many women in the sex industry are sexual abuse survivors is because such trauma often results in a woman feeling a "separation" from her own physical body due to having such abuse inflicted upon her.

For example, it was not uncommon to hear a woman in the business feel as if she were empowering herself by capitalizing on her sexuality, and given the fact that things such as "virginity" or her "sexual body" were abused and taken advantage of before, using her body for money was in a sick way, "taking control" of what happened. Though to many it may not make sense, the actuality is that for an abused woman, her mentality may be that her body was never hers to begin with, so using it for money was taking control back and using it to further her own ends instead. However, I always felt, and still feel that I used stripping as not only a way to capitalize on and take control of a body I had never felt ownership of, but I also chose the profession as a way to subconsciously continue the abuse that I felt I "deserved."

At age 21 I was involved in my first really serious love relationship, something that was and is still very challenging for me due to my trust issues with men. During this time I was working a great deal as a model and travelling all over the world for shoots and events.

It was during this time, at 21 years old, that I lost my best friend, Derek MacQuarrie, who was my high school sweetheart, first love, and the young man who had taught me how to begin trusting men. About 2 months after his passing I became the victim of a violent rape by a photographer I had been sent to shoot with for my agency.

Though I had dealt with so much sexual abuse in the past, what was the most crushing for me this time around was that I blamed myself for allowing it to happen as I had promised myself that after all my childhood abuse I would never allow myself to be victimized again. For 6 months I waited patiently to ensure that I did not contract HIV or AIDS from the assault. My relationship eventually ended due to the fact I was so emotionally shut off from the death of my best friend and the trauma of my rape, and so I fell deeper into my addiction.

During my 20's I struggled with my addiction, in and out of meetings and rehab, and had been admitted for drug overdose. When things were good, I would have several months, and at one time up to a year and half at a time that I would maintain sobriety, but in the end I would always relapse. I continued on as an addict throughout my college years and was able to somehow graduate with honors in 2009, despite the fact that at this point my addictions had spun out of control to where I no longer was speaking to most of my family and had cut off anyone and everyone who had an issue with or dared to confront me about my addiction.

In the late summer of 2009 I awakened after hitting "rock bottom." It was September of 2009 and I had just returned to Orange County where I lived after a 30-day drug binge and non-stop party stay in Vegas. My friends in Vegas had held an intervention for me a few days before as they had not realized how bad my addiction was until my extended time visiting and I left Las Vegas to return home for a few days as I was angry with them for confronting me about "my problem.".

At this point I was spending thousands a month to feed my addiction, my credit cards were maxed out, bills were going unpaid, my health was deteriorating and my physical body was already shutting down with kidney infections, kidney stones, sinus infections, anemia, malnutrition, and my life was falling apart. Upon returning to OC, I was running errands and going on 2 days of no sleep and almost killed a family crossing at a pedestrian crosswalk, in broad daylight, but instead nearly totaled my car driving onto the sidewalk to avoid hitting them with my vehicle. Horrified and scared by what had happened I went home and binged on cocaine. That night I remember trying to lay in bed to sleep, my heart was beating so rapidly it started to scare me, and breathing became difficult as I felt like I had a ton of bricks on my chest. As I tried to move my body was so weak and felt paralyzed and I realized I may be about to overdose. I remember the anxiety and sadness I felt as I thought to myself, "I am going to die tonight, alone in my home. I haven't spoken to my family in months and my friends all have no idea what city or state I am even in. It may be days until they find my body, and when they perform the autopsy my parents will know I died of a drug overdose." I remember praying for my life, promising that if I made it through the night I would stop using for good.

When I awoke the next day I looked in the mirror and realized I had no idea who I was anymore. The gauntness of my face, the pale color of my skin, the dead stillness of my eyes; it was awful. I called one of my best friends from recovery who I had not spoken to in months and he took me to my first meeting. Though I had made efforts towards my sobriety before, this time was different. I realized that I had been given two chances at life when I should have died from overdose, and knew that would not have another chance if I made the wrong choice.

The first several months of my recovery were the worst both physically and emotionally. However, as time went on I began to improve. During my recovery I was forced to begin facing the real reasons I used drugs, and for the first time in my life I truly began to heal and address the issues and pain I had been using drugs to avoid for so long. It wasn't until I was about 6 months into my sobriety that I was able to truly accept and face the fact that my childhood sexual abuse was the reason I had turned to drugs to begin with. Making the decision to truly face the pain I carried inside was terrifying for me, as I knew it would be a long and difficult journey. Little did I know however, that the source of my greatest pain would later become the fuel for my success, and the inspiration for my life's purpose to educate and empower others.

As I continued to evolve in my recovery I returned to fitness as a way to deal with the depression that came with detox and to rebuild my body, which had withered away to nothing as a result of years of drug abuse. Making my body stronger and rebuilding what years of drug abuse had nearly destroyed was empowering for me and eventually bodybuilding became my passion, leading me to where I am today.

In 2011 I entered my first Bikini and Figure Competitions and won my height class and the overall at my very first Figure Competition, an accomplishment that was very meaningful to me as the strong, fit, and healthy, 5'2" 116lb body I had built was a huge difference from the sick and malnourished 98lb I had during the peak of my addiction. Though I no longer compete, I am still very active in Fitness and work as a coach for other athletes competing in Men's Physique, Women's Bikini, and Women's Figure.

Though I am now living a fulfilling life that I love and am passionate about, while helping others to achieve a healthier lifestyle, I am far from accomplishing what I believe my life purpose to be. And though I continue to face challenges and have faced far more hardship than I could even begin to write in this chapter, I refuse to allow anything to break me or destroy me. I know and realize that if I made it through what I did, it was for a reason, and that I am strong because of it. I believe that nothing can break you unless you allow it to, but it took me years of self-inflicted suffering and addiction to realize how true that statement is.

As I write this I am amidst a very difficult Domestic Violence case against my recent boyfriend who became physical at the end of our relationship and tried to choke and strangle me during our breakup. However, despite the emotional turmoil I am in due to recent circumstances, returning to drugs or self-destructive behaviors is not even something I would consider and I am remaining strong and hopeful. Just like my abusers, I will not allow him to break me or rob me of the life I deserve to live.

If there is anything that I hold to be firm and true it is that an individual has the power to make the decision as to whether or not they will allow something bad that has happened to destroy them, or if they will use it to make them stronger. I am living proof of the choice to live as an unbreakable survivor and not as a victim. I spent years of my life in self-pity and angry at the world for cards I was dealt, but I no longer allow my experiences to imprison me.

In order to continue to deal with the pain that still lingers from my experiences, I remind myself daily that I was given the battles I was given because I was strong enough to handle them, and I know in my heart that someday I will be a driving force in creating greater awareness for difficult issues such as Domestic Violence, Sexual Abuse, Rape, Incest, and Drug Addiction. I believe that it is through sharing our story that we heal ourselves and empower others who have experienced similar things, and I hope that my story will help other women to see that they are not alone, that there is hope, and that no matter what has happened, you deserve love and happiness and can pursue the life of your dreams and attain success.

I believe I was put on this Earth and given the challenges I was given to someday help the world in a grand scale. I know I am still alive, against all odds, because my purpose in this world is not yet fulfilled. Someday I will stand before thousands sharing my story, empowering others and heading foundations and charities that provide resources for those that have been victimized.

I now know I am unbreakable, and hope to help others find the same strength and courage within themselves to guide them through whatever challenges life throws their way.

Carla Maria Cadotte
I'm a 5'1 Filipina Muscle Barbie: NPC National Figure Athlete & Competition Prep Coach, Playboy & Penthouse Model, Fitness Model / NSCA CPT.

Nothing Comes Easy...
But The Grind is Worth it
by Heidi Cannon

It's very true to life, nothing comes easy. For some people, however, they seem to have it all, and I'm thinking to myself how the heck did they get where they're at and why the heck wasn't that me!!! Of course that's just me being jealous. But placing that aside, I can totally relate to this motto because it's one in which I try to live by. I also feel extremely blessed to be surrounded by a loving and supportive husband, family and close friends who are the positive influences in my life.

From a young adult, I've always been active, even a "tom boy" as some people call me. Just about every sport out there I love to try, and am up for experiencing anything new or extreme. And, if I really like something, I work my butt off to get good at it.

When I was 13 years old, my parents enrolled me into martial arts, which was a smart move on their part! After going twice, I was hooked! I had amazing teachers who instilled in me lifelong values such as respect, dedication, commitment and hard work. I also met so many nice people who are still friends to this day. I trained 3-5 times a week, and ultimately achieved my Black Belt at 18. Later that same year my team was going to Melbourne Australia to compete in the World Martial Arts Games. I wanted to go and compete so badly and to be part of the team but didn't get picked. I was totally crushed, Weeks later it was decided that if any one wanted to go they could pay their own way and come. So, I decided to go, and much to the surprise of my teammates and others, I competed in two competitions and won gold medals in both.

During my time down under, I discovered the Australian Stunt Academy in Brisbane Australia. I thought to myself...I love to be in front of people and I'm really good at sports -- this is a perfect fit!! I can act and do my own stunts! The following year, I enrolled in the course and loved it, learning all the stunt person's basics from being lit on fire, to getting hit by a car, to repelling off cliffs and even scuba diving. I was so excited and pumped to get home and eventually move to Vancouver and start pursuing my dreams.

Shortly after I returned home there was an advertisement from Universal Studios California looking for stuntwomen. This was my big break, or so I thought, so I flew to Burbank California with my Mom and went to the try-outs where I found out I was one of hundreds competing for the same role. On the second round, I was "chopped." Again, another blow to my ego, and yet I wasn't ready to give up. I was determined to move to Vancouver and start my new stunt/acting gig.

I think I was under the total illusion that by moving to Vancouver I would get "noticed" or "discovered" and "bam," I would break into the movie scene. Nothing could have been farther from the truth. Early on, I found out I had HUGE competition, and it required me finding an agent that believed in me. I foolishly thought they would see me and go "wow", you're "it". Ha ha! I did get an agent and started going to numerous auditions. At the time I also was holding down a full-time job and needed to give a day's notice to take time off in the middle of the day to go to an audition. Luckily for me I had an understanding boss.

If I wanted to stay on top of my game I had to start taking acting classes again. So after work, twice a week, I would drive 45 minutes to acting class, which was 2 hours long, then take the 45 minute drive back home. On the other "free" nights, I worked out at the local gym where all the working stunt performers trained, trying to get my face known.

I got a call from my agent who told me she had booked me a gig to ride a motorcycle for a Macy's commercial. I was so excited I nearly threw up. I can remember showing up on set and seeing my name on the door of the trailer I was meant to stay in while shooting, and thinking this is it! I'm on a roll now!. Well...that was short-lived because I didn't get booked for anything else until 3 months later.

As time went on I started to get a bit disheartened with the endless auditions and nothing to show for it. And, I was noticing that some of the stunt roles were being given to other girls that weren't necessarily stunt performers. I began to see a totally different side to the acting/stunt world and I asked myself "why am I putting in so much effort on all levels and draining my bank account for what?" I can't say that it was all bad and it was pretty cool seeing myself in a television commercial or in a television series.

It was time for me to move on and find another outlet and a new focus. This is when I decided to take a course in esthetics - something I had always been fascinated in, and it gave me an opportunity to broaden my career path. While there, I was very fortunate to meet so many great people that were like me who were in their later 20's trying to change their career paths as well.

It was during this time that I used to frequent a coffee shop on our lunch hour, and the guy who owned the shop was huge!!! He had massive biceps and triceps. He must be a bodybuilder. Sure enough I was right. He replied back saying that he competed in bodybuilding. Sweet! Thinking to myself, how hard could it be? I've been lit on fire, I've achieved my black belt, jumped my dirt bike 100 feet, I'm sure I could figure out how to put a routine together and walk around in a bikini.

After watching numerous YouTube videos of women doing fitness routines, to train me for my very first show I hired the help of my two good friends who were heavily involved in the sport. Fortunately I had a dance background – yes, this "tom boy" loves to dance (years of practice and taking multiple dance classes in belly dance and other forms of dance) and who knew, was not too bad at it lol!

I decided to incorporate my love of belly dance into my routine and learned how to do the fitness holds and poses that were required. For 4 months, every other day I practiced putting a routine together and worked out with my trainer, and went to the gym 3 times a week.

The morning of the first show I was so sick. I had never before put my body through such a rigorous training schedule and strict diet plan in all my life! Because of being so active, I had never had to diet before and ate and drank whatever I wanted. Now it was totally different.

Knowing that I wanted to win more than anything, my competitive side kicked in. Everything I had trained and sacrificed for came down to that moment. I got on the stage and went for it - nailing all my holds and dance moves - definitely a huge accomplishment for me, and I ended up placing second in my first show. Oh was I ever pumped! I was on a roll.

Two weeks later, I entered the WBFF show, placing in the top three. Believe me, I was on top of the world! I thought to myself why not do one more this year. The show was 6 weeks later and I had fallen off the strict diet plan completely. Thinking I would be able to get back onto the stage in top shape in a matter of 2 weeks was impossible. I placed 5th in BC for fitness but I knew in my heart I could have achieved better. I was totally down on myself and was eating everything in sight. But then I decided to change to a realistic attitude and commit myself again to striving for that number one spot in a sensible way. For the next six months I trained and the following June I trained for the WBFF Vancouver Championships, where came in first place and won my pro card. I had done it!!!!!!

My philosophy in life is to truly believe in yourself, and through hard work and effort, visualize yourself accomplishing whatever goal you're striving for. And, if one door closes, another door will open for you.

Everything in God's time. Do your best and help everyone else along the way, and be grateful for each day that you do have.

And remember: nothing comes easy...but the grind is worth it!

Heidi Cannon

I'm a Magnum sponsored athlete, WBFF pro fitness model, published professional belly dancer and stunt performer.

How to Rise From The Ashes
by Phoenix Carnevale

Throughout her life Phoenix Carnevale, a nationally recognized Mixed Martial Arts journalist, on camera personality, fight commentator, fitness expert, and fighter, has remained true to her name. Like the legendary bird, which rises from the ashes, she has never been afraid to meet challenges and create opportunities for herself in her multifaceted and ever-expanding career. Phoenix's passion for personal growth, good story telling and shedding light on human potential is the fire behind her drive.

Brooklyn born, and a New Yorker in every sense of the word, Phoenix was raised in a single parent household and primarily looked after by her older brother David. By spending her time with her brother she became the ultimate tomboy. Comic books, action movies and Bruce Lee quotes all became staples of her upbringing. Her obsession with martial arts started at a young age, but she wasn't able to afford lessons until she was an adult. But instead of giving up on her dreams as soon as she had the opportunity she pursued her lifelong passion and made her dreams into a reality.

Phoenix was able to finally fulfill her childhood dream of studying Martial Arts when she signed up for Seido Karate. At Seido Karate, under the strict tutelage of Kaicho Nakamura, Phoenix gained a deep understanding of eastern wisdom and philosophy. Seido helped her develop her interest in traditional martial arts and gave her a foundation for her training. Looking to expand her training, Phoenix headed to Gleason's Gym in Brooklyn New York and trained under MMA boxing coach Mike Smith. At Gleason's Phoenix sparred and trained alongside professional MMA athletes, boxing world champions and some of the best fighters in the business. Befriending these pros helped Phoenix gain an up close understanding of these remarkable athletes, and an appreciation for their craft.

Phoenix was athletic, but she had never focused on her conditioning before, and she was looking for more ways to improve herself, and her physical condition. She hit the gym and in less than a year transformed her body. This new passion to lead a healthy lifestyle for herself caused her to want to help others in their own fitness journeys. Phoenix began her successful and ever-growing career in the health and wellness industry. She began teaching a variety of fun and innovative classes at such clubs as Equinox, NYHRC and NYSC as well as teaching wellness seminars at universities around New York State. She has been featured locally on FOX news, ABC news, CBS news, NY1, and the CW11 morning show, as well as national programs such as Lifetime Womens' Next Stop New You, Spike TV's Rocky Marathon. American Latino TV highlighted Phoenix 's career in order to inspire Latinos to live a healthier life. She has also appeared in numerous fitness publications.

However, during her boxing training Phoenix seriously injured her foot and needed months of rehab. This was a large setback for her, and all of her hard work seemed to be slipping away. Frustrated about being unable to compete in the Golden Gloves, instead of giving up and turning her back on her passion, Phoenix decided to make the most out her her time off of training. She began reading everything and anything there was on all things martial arts. She was so involved in her self guided studies that her friends began to refer to her as a martial arts encyclopedia. She began her Martial Arts journalism career.

While doing her research she came across Muay Thai boxing and the name Kru Phil Nurse. Thai Boxing seemed to be the perfect blend that Phoenix was looking for, all the spirituality and philosophy of Karate mixed with the toughness she loved about boxing. Despite the fact that she was in physical therapy and couldn't train Phoenix decided to go to Phil's school, The Wat, in New York City. Meeting Phil was kismet. He became the most influential person in her martial arts career, and ultimately in her life. She spent afternoons sitting watching him teach, and this observation ultimately showed her how to teach, and how to see as well. She listened closely to his teachings while still in recovery and once she was fully able she immediately started to train at The Wat. Eventually she began fighting with Phil as her coach. She is a devoted friend and student to him, and he has helped her realize her full potential.

Phoenix has now used her extensive knowledge and passion for martial arts into a thriving MMA journalism career, and has been contributing to many martial arts journalism venues, both writing articles and interviewing fighters. She has hosted and produced segments on Inside Martial Arts, which quickly gained her a cult following. The segments were later showcased on Black belt TV. Phoenix can also be seen monthly on ESPN U's sports show UNITE giving a complete analysis on UFC's up and coming main events. Phoenix has interviewed martial arts legends and champions such as Cung Le, Matt Serra, Gina Carano, Chael Sonnen, and Ronda Rousey. In addition Phoenix co-produced, "At the Wat" a series of sit-down interviews with professional fighters focusing on MMA stars - athletes such as UFC champion Georges St. Pierre, former lightweight champion Frankie Edgar, UFC light heavyweight champion Jon Jones.

As her interest in being on camera grew Phoenix spread her wings and took to the stage, performing in theatre groups around the country. She has currently performed and written for a variety of stand up comedy clubs such as Gotham Comedy Club and NY Comedy Club.

Most recently Eddie Cuello of Take On Productions invited Phoenix to co-commentate the Muay Thai shows. She jumped at the opportunity, becoming the color commentator for several shows including Battle at Bally's 1 and 2, Take On's 8 Man tournament and Muay Thai at the Mecca 1 & 2, the first time Muay Thai kickboxing was ever presented at Madison Square Garden. This led to other commentating gigs both in New York and abroad, including commentating on Sky Active Networks Muay Thai World Series and Fighting Force Championship in Bournemouth, England. Take On recently shot a pilot for MSG networks with Phoenix hosting and giving color commentary.

At this point in her life and career, Phoenix is concentrating on on-camera hosting, MMA journalism and performing. She is working to produce all-inclusive Martial Arts-related media and materials so that others can profit from and enjoy the beauty and power of these disciplines. Phoenix will no doubt continue to rise in all of her varied pursuits.

Phoenix Carnevale
I'm a Martial Arts obsessed journalist, fight commentator, show host and comedian.

Katie's Journey to Happiness & Health
by Katie Cates

Hey there! I'm Katie Cates a mother of 1 and wife to one amazing man. My insecurities started back in middle school. One little comment "You shouldn't wear those pants, your cellulite shows" ruined me for years to come.

During my high school years I passed up just about the entire summer. I was not going to be seen in shorts, skirts, dresses or a bathing suit. I played sports in high school and hated every minute of it, not because of the sport but because of the shorts. Track and Volleyball had such short shorts and that was literally all I could think about while on the court or on the track. As a young woman you associate cellulite with being fat and feeling fat can lead to depression or even eating disorders. I suppose I was lucky enough to have never had an eating disorder, but I did and still do suffer from what I claim as minor depression or anxiety over the littlest things.

Now, lets fast forward to early stages of marriage. This is where the insecurities came out in full force. Nothing will make a woman feel more insecure about her looks than knowing what a great guy she has, but not knowing how 'forever' it would be. My husband would tell me over and over how much he loved me the way I was and how he supported me in any decision I made, but the problem was still present. It wasn't until I was pregnant that I gained any motivation to change my ways. During my pregnancy I gained 40 pounds and weighed in at 201 lbs. the day of delivery with a baby weighing a tiny 6 lbs. 7 oz. It wasn't until delivery that I knew I had my work cut out for me.

After my son, Layton was born it was time for some major goal setting and keeping the motivation going! My goals were small, achievable and each goal had a date attached to it. My biggest goal was to be back in my pre-pregnancy clothing in 9 months or less. There are several women who do this in a much shorter amount of time, but it took me 9 months to gain my 40 lbs., so I gave myself 9 months to lose it. I am very happy to say I lost my 40 lbs. in 7 months! After my 1st goal, each goal became more 'fine-tuned' so to speak. Each week I would set goals and some would be as small as run 1 mile a day, while others may be eat clean 95% of the time. Other goals were to limit alcohol from my diet. Each goal helped me reach my current physical state.

After losing my initial 40 pounds I was tightly in a size 11/12 jean and weighing in at 160 pounds. Motherhood isn't an easy job and my body didn't bounce back into place without a fight. Being a new mom in a town with no friends and family was hard enough, but being all those things and trying to make time for myself, my fitness and learn how to eat for the body I wanted was not an easy task at hand. I had good days, bad days and really awful days. With each new day I encountered I also became stronger, not only physically but mentally as well. You see I wasn't born with the genetics of a fitness model or any model. I knew the body I wanted was going to be hard work, but I didn't know it would be that hard.

5 months postpartum I became overly sensitive to just about anything or anyone with an opinion other than mine. I cried all day and I would cry at night while my husband was asleep. It wasn't until one night that I woke my husband up and asked him to just sit there and listen to me, to not speak, to not judge and to not laugh at me. I began to tell him how I was thinking about self-harm and how I understand why people do such things. I could see the fear in his eyes as they began wandering around on my body. I quickly told him that I didn't hurt myself, but was afraid of what may happen if I didn't get help soon. My husband was amazing through the whole process and even asked if I wanted him to

call the doctor for me, but I wanted to reach out for help on my own to prove that I was strong enough to want better for myself, my husband and my son. The following morning I called my OBGYN and began a prescription for antidepressants. In the beginning I felt like a failure because I needed help, but soon after I realized how strong of a woman I was for reaching out for help. It takes courage to not feel like you are a failure when asking for help. Postpartum was my biggest setback, but also my biggest achievement. Dealing with postpartum set my standards high because I knew if I could get past this I could get past anything.

Three months after reaching out for help I was going strong! My workouts had increased and my nutrition was becoming easier. At this time I decided I was ready for a bigger challenge and ready to accomplish some real goals. I contacted my great friend and mentor CJ Woodruff about a custom meal plan and custom workout plan. Once I received my plans I joined a gym for the very first time at the age of Twenty-Four. I had no idea what I was doing in there, but knew if I wanted it bad enough I needed to start my research.

Every day that week I went into the gym with my plan in hand and cell phone in the other. I had to Googled every move because I was new to weightlifting and the gym. It was funny now thinking back how I had to watch videos over and over to make sure I was doing things correct. I will never forget the feeling of walking into the gym to sign up for the very first time. It was like going to school on the first day, a sense of excitement and nervousness. Once I found my groove in the weight room it wasn't long after that CJ gave me a shout and asked if I would like to attend his school, PFTA (Personal Trainer School).

The thought of going 'back to school' after 8 years was a bit intimidating and took a lot of thought. I discussed the opportunity with my husband and of course he was supportive of my decision. Becoming a personal trainer and sports nutritionist was never on my list of things to be when I grew up, Ha-Ha. It had actually never crossed my mind, not even while losing weight, but once the idea was put in front of me that's all I could think about. I thought about it every day until I started class in 2011. December 2011 I was handed two certifications, CSN & CPT. I was beyond blessed and thankful for CJ and all that he did for me. Having these two certifications now allowed me to help other women who were struggling as I did. I could now offer education and motivation!

As I sit here today in 2013 I look back at all I have accomplished and have done with no college degree or classes on business. I worked my way from high school, to working full time, marriage, being a mom, battling my weight to gaining my certifications to now running and operating a business helping women and men lose weight and stay motivated. As the years move past me I would like to achieve notoriety in just about any fitness magazine and would love to one day be able to travel and speak to others about weight loss and what they can do to help get on track and stay there.

My job here isn't complete—it's just the beginning.

Katie Cates

I'm inspiring women & men of all ages to get fit & healthy in a fun and carefree manner!

Passion is Everything
by Lori & Michelle Corso

Drive. Determination. Persistence. Passion. Working hard. Sweat. Sacrifice.

Some words that come to mind when we think of what it means to be an entrepreneur. The strongest word that truly means everything is PASSION.

- You need to have passion to drive you.
- You need passion to get you up off the couch and go DO the work.
- You need passion to keep you going even when you run into problems and hurdles.
- Passion gets you up every morning.
- Passion energizes you to accomplish your tasks for the day.
- Passion helps you overcome challenges you will face daily.
- Without passion it will be impossible to make it.

We wake up everyday being grateful for being able to work for ourselves. Yes we have had to give up a lot, make sacrifice after sacrifice. Do we regret any of it? NO! Because every problem we ran into, we learned. Every time we made a mistake, we learned. Every new opportunity came to us because we kept going.

We always looked at the bigger picture. But we also focused on the present tasks, while pushing hard to reach our goals. Staying focused on the main end goal is key. You will make many mistakes along the way but focusing on the end goal will keep that inner passion going.

Once you decided what you are passionate about, you are granting yourself to design your own life. Align your passions with your desires to become incredibly empowering.

We are sharing 5 basic tips we feel are important in taking the steps to following your passion to make it a reality.

5 tips to help you be passionate about your work:

1. You have to DECIDE to be passionate. Once you make the decision to be passionate, then you will have the drive to do it. Saying it out loud to yourself helps get things going. Saying it out loud to others makes it REAL. Choosing passion you are deciding to be hopeful, cheerful and find things that feed your flame. So find that deep meaning and there you will get your passion.

2. You need WILL. Do you have the willpower to survive? Having WILL is the key to unlocking your desire, your passion. After you admit that you're passionate, next comes WILL. The WILL to do it. The WILL not to stop. Your WILL come across times when your passion fails, your WILL takes its place until passion returns. A new breakthrough will come and your passion will again shine.

3. You will need a plan. Okay so you have the passion and the will to do whatever it takes, now what? You need a plan. A road map so to speak. Write out how you are going to do it. Write out your goals, then the steps to reach those goals. Make short and long term goals. Once you have the plan, go take action. Face your fear. Believe in your dream. Work hard each day to make it a reality.

4. Surround yourself with inspiration. The key to staying positive is surrounding yourself with positivity. Connect with like-minded people. Connect will people that help, inspire, and motivate you. People that remind you that no matter what, YOU can do it. If there is anything in your life that is bringing you down leave it behind. Don't let others convince you that following your passion is not practical.

5. You need to visualize achieving your dream. Need to picture yourself reaching your final goal. The more real you paint the picture

in your mind the better. If you truly see yourself doing what you are passionate about then you will achieve it. Remember the mind is a powerful tool. Use it to your advantage. Visualize yourself reaching your dream everyday, as often as you can. When we feel down, go and picture yourself where you want to be. Focus on that.

Those five tips are just the foundation to start following your dream with passion. Remember even highly successful business owners have experienced failure or a setback a few times on their journey to success.

We went through several failures during our road to where we are today! Being passionate about our dreams is the one thing that kept us going. We are passionate about helping others live their best life. We are passionate about making healthy recipes, spreading our love of fitness, and showing others how to enjoy their BEST life.

Continue to pursue your passion. You have the right to do so. Keep yourself focused and motivated each day. Find that passion in everything you do! Set your goals and pursue them relentlessly. Being women business owners means so much to us, as we get to inspire, help, motivate, and be a FRIEND to others. And this is where our passion comes from helping others!

We help motivated, beautiful, strong, confident women to become even more confident and beautiful by helping them become the BEST versions of themselves.

We are passionate twin sisters, best friends, and business partners. We are chefs, writers, and authors of Purelytwins.com. Two big passions, we have are food and fitness, and we are honored to have achieved our dreams. We published our first cookbook, Purely Classic Recipes, and created an online home workout program Purely Fit Life. We are driven to help people live healthier, happier, and active lifestyles.

Our passion never stops. Yours shouldn't either. Remember passion is the fuel that can drive you towards the realization of your dreams. Passion helps you live a purposeful life. When you live with purpose and passion, great things happen!

Lori & Michelle Corso

We are twin sisters. Chefs. Trainers. Fitfluential ambassadors. Multi-passionate entrepreneurs. Bloggers.

Don't Tell Me I Can't
by Dr. AnnMaria De Mars

"B****, I will break your f****** arm!" is perhaps not the best statement with which to begin an inspirational essay. However, it is a good summary of my attitude when I competed in judo.

Unlike timed events, where a clock determines who wins, judo is a 'judged sport'; a referee decides on the score. My opponent looked like she ought to be on a Wheaties box. I looked like I ought to be on a wanted poster. If it came down to a decision, who do you think would win?"

A great judo player, Pat Burris, gave me sage advice:

"Go for the armbar. Even if the referee doesn't score it, if you break her arm, for the rest of the match, you're fighting a one-armed woman. If you can't beat a one-armed woman, babe, you deserve to lose."

I refused to accept that my success was in anyone's hands but my own. Like many of my competitors' arms, I took that rule and broke it.

I always wondered if maybe there was a week during my school years when they got all of the girls in the room and gave them The Rules. If there was a week like that, I must have been out sick and missed it because all of my life nearly everyone around me has acted as if there was this set of rules:

Your physical appearance will never match up to what it should be.

It makes a difference what clothes you wear.

Girls aren't good at math.

No man wants a woman who comes home from practice soaking wet with sweat.

Women can't be as successful as men in business, because they have children to raise.

Don't say anything that might upset people.

I have heard these lines all of my life. Even though I'm probably the oldest author in this book, I still don't understand these attitudes any better than when I was a child. Throughout my life, I repeatedly have been asked:

"Why can't you be like everybody else?"

"Why can't you just accept that there are some things you CAN'T do?"

"Why do you always act like the rules don't apply to you?"

"Just who do you think you are?"

Fifty years ago, I couldn't accept that schools had boys' sports but not girls' sports. Thirty years ago, I couldn't accept that women couldn't be engineers. Today, I can't accept that grandmothers can't be CEO of a successful technology start-up, especially not in gaming.

Who do I think I am? I've been a world judo champion, engineer, professor, statistical consultant, CEO and author. All of my life, I've answered outraged questioners the same way, "I'm me."

Twenty years ago, a student at the college where I was teaching wrote me a heart-felt note saying that he was going to graduate in a few weeks and he felt he really did not fit into his small North Dakota town. He asked if I had any advice to offer that might help him find a direction in life. The answer I gave him then is the one I would give today.

All of my life, I have tried to live by my own rules. I cannot guarantee that this will make you happy, but it has worked for me, and if you are asking me this question, it will probably work for you.

The second rule that I refused to accept was that women must be continually evaluating their looks - in parts, no less. It takes me 15 minutes to get ready to go anywhere. The only time I look at myself in the mirror is when I'm brushing my hair and teeth in the morning. If I give any thought to my appearance, it is this, "I look fine." Then, I go about my day. I have never for one second thought that my nose was too big, my breasts too small or thought of myself in any way other than a whole person.

I am sure I developed a healthy body image from participating in sports most of my life. I started judo at age 12 because it was one of the few sports in the small town where I lived that girls were allowed to join. (Yes, in those days before Title IX legislation required programs accepting federal funds to provide equal opportunities for males and females, many organizations had rules against women joining the team.) When, thanks to Title IX again, my college started a track team for women, I joined that.

It wasn't just the sports in which I participated but the type of sport. Unlike predominantly female sports, such as gymnastics and ice-skating, looks play no part in winning when it came to judo or track. No one cares about your outfit, your sparkly make-up or how your hair is styled. It's 100 percent what you can do.

The third rule I decided didn't apply to me was that there is one path to success. As a competitor, I didn't have the funding that my competitors did to travel around the world. However, when I was an undergraduate, I applied for the year-abroad program at my university. Since my scholarship money could be used toward that, I was able to live and train in Japan at Waseda University my junior year and still graduate from college when I was 19.

The fourth rule I have flaunted all of my life, and the one that outrages people the most, is that women aren't allowed the same choices as men. After starting a male sport at 12, I went to college and took lots of classes that were predominantly male - Calculus, computer programming, and mathematical statistics. As a statistician, I can't help but see a relationship here. Many women I know who grew up in judo went on to have careers in traditionally male-dominated fields. I think perhaps these women became comfortable being the only female in a room. When they saw opportunities in fields like engineering, they were not held back the fact that all the others pursuing those opportunities were men.

Act 2: I want to replace math class with a game.

So here, I am now, founder and CEO of 7 Generation Games. No one can be farther from the Silicon Valley stereotype of a high-tech startup founder than me. I didn't go to Stanford or an Ivy League school and dropout. I attended Washington University in St. Louis, an excellent college in the Midwest. I graduated, then went on to get two masters degrees and a Ph.D. I'm not twenty-something. I'm fifty-something. I'm not single. I have a husband, four daughters and two granddaughters.

I've wanted to create a game to teach kids math ever since I got my first Macintosh computer back in 1984. As you have deduced by now, my success in life hasn't been due to my sweet personality and willingness to abide by the rules. If I had not been good at math, I am quite sure I'd be in Chino Women's Prison right now. Because I was good at two things, first judo and then math, I received a pass on a lot of my worse qualities. People took me under their wing and mentored me.

How did I get good at math? The same way I got good at judo. I did a lot of it. If there was a game that included math, I reasoned, and kids liked it enough to play it a lot, they would get better, too. So, I decided to make a game like that and developed one that would appeal to both students who liked math and to students who hated school but just liked computer games.

At angel investor meetings, it was pretty clear the type of founder that was being sought. Some were honest enough to state bluntly that "younger people are digital natives, they understand the market" or "young people don't have children to go home to, so they can put in the hours necessary for a startup."

Confronted with this, I did what I've always done. I skipped the standard path. We received $550,000 in grant funds, $21,000 in Kickstarter funds and we already have thousands of users, as our game is in twenty schools this fall who have agreed to be test sites. Kids who play our game are scoring better on standardized tests than kids who just read their textbooks and do worksheets - and they're having a good time.

What have I learned in the end? That you don't have to accept the rules other people write for you. Whatever it is that you want to achieve, work until you get it. Don't let anybody tell you that you can't. Never give up. Never let anyone stop you, even if it means you have to break an arm or two along the way.

Dr. AnnMaria De Mars
I'm a PhD, CEO, world champion and mom.

Finding Your Inner Strength
by Karen Gallagher

Looking back on the past thirty years, I can honestly say that I have been very blessed in my life. As a little girl I grew up on a beautiful hobby farm, I road my own horse daily and when I was not mucking around on the farm you would find me at the local rink figure skating. Even though I was an only child I was surrounded with a loving family and many supportive friends. I was considered a little shy and introverted (still am a bit!). I had a big heart and I loved to help others. Remembering those years, everything seemed so perfect to me.

Life in general seemed normal to me; I was young and excited for the future! I went away to school, met my husband, fell in love, started my fitness career and assumed my life was going to play out precisely like a playbook…I would get married, buy a house, have a family, grow old together and live happily ever after. After 18 years together our love bond broke and so did my heart. What we had together would never be restored. I never once thought I would ever be sitting here today sharing my story about the ending of my marriage and loss of love.

I truly believe that in life we are meant to take certain pathways in order to learn and grow as individuals. When I look back on my marriage and our 18-year relationship I can honestly say that I'm blessed to have experienced everything that I did, including the heartbreak. Being in love is extremely special and it can sometimes be rare to find. I was very lucky to have found someone to share this unique bond with and to be married. As well, I was fortunate to have experienced the hardships over the later part of my marriage because I realize now how it has challenged me to learn more about myself and to grow stronger.

One of the most challenging obstacles as a trainer and motivator is the pressure to appear seamless everyday, all day and in every aspect of your life. Sometimes fitness professionals are perceived this way because people believe if we look great then we MUST also have the perfect life to go along with it. At first, I felt embarrassed to share my story with others because I feared that people would judge and think less of me. I didn't want to show people my vulnerable side, the side that was weak and broken. I wanted to still be perceived as being strong both mentally and physically. I used to tell myself, "You can fake this until it is all over and no one will ever know. You are a ROCK!" Recently, I have come to realize that I need to be real and true to myself by sharing my story. Most importantly, I want to share with women how my most challenging life experience has empowered me and how fitness was my savior.

I remember the day like it was yesterday, the day my relationship ended. I felt like a MAC truck hit me. I cried for what seemed like days until I virtually had no more tears left to shed. I lost the love of my life – I was devastated. I felt a cold emptiness in my heart. There were some days when I did not even want to get out of bed, days were I could not eat or sleep. I felt lonely, unwanted and unloved, fearful, anxious, defeated and like a failure. After two years of putting all my energy into salvaging my marriage, I finally felt like I hit rock bottom. I lost my partner in life and as well somewhere along the way I lost myself. I realized that during this entire downward spiral I became this unrecognizable person – I lost my self-esteem, my purpose and passion for life, and the sense of who I truly was. I just wanted the old Karen back.

Then I got angry. I felt betrayed by my husband and by life itself. I felt angry that I was in such a negative place and that I wasted two years of my life which I would never get back. I felt overwhelmed and exhausted from the emotional roller coaster I was on. Behind all my anger were fears such as: "Will I be alone for the rest of my life?" "How will I support myself?" "Am I worthy of being loved?" I drove myself crazy with negative thoughts and energy and it was sucking the life out of me. I knew that I had to face my fears and look after myself. I made a choice to be positive, surround myself with loving and supportive people, love and treat myself with respect, and keep healthy.

The end of a love relationship can be very painful and I can relate to so many women who have experienced it and have struggled to find themselves again. What is important to know is that you are not alone and it is possible to find your inner strength again in order to put the relationship in the past and to move forward in life. You want to thrive during this challenging time, not just survive it. You need to believe that you are more than enough, you are worthy and you deserve the best. I see challenge as a gift in life, without challenge new opportunities cannot arise and therefore we are not forced to face our fears and grow as humans. I want to share with you how I found my inner strength and how it has empowered me to create a new pathway of dreams.

Stop Blaming and Forgive

Putting the blame on yourself and your spouse will only cause more harm and hurt. I knew that beating myself up over what could or should have been was an endless battle. I acknowledged and accepted what I did and what I did not do and simply learned from it and just let it go. Forgiveness is also so important in moving forward, you need to forgive yourself and your partner in order to recover. What is in the past is the past and holding onto negative feelings will only keep you in a negative place.

Become clear on what you want in Life - Write a Wish List

How do you envision your life? What do you truly want to experience and feel? Write a wishlist of what you want for each area of your life. I focused on these areas: career, family, health, partner in life and friends. For each, I listed every quality and how I wanted to feel. When you start focusing on what you do want, the quicker you become to receiving it in your life.

Take Care of YOU!

Focus on your body and how you want to feel. Work on areas that you want to improve on or areas you want to maintain. Make fitness a part of your life. What truly saved me was my passion and commitment to health and fitness. It provided me with positive energy that empowered me to keep strong and confident. I had a purpose to get up in the morning, a reason to keep strong and a reason to move forward in a positive direction. For once in my life fitness became a huge support to save me and not something I had to do for a sport, competition, shoot or for anyone else, it was for ME. It was the catalyst that kept me strong physically and mentally and it has opened doors to possibilities and relationships in which I would have never encountered if I made the choice to remain down.

Live in the Moment

By living in the moment, you are not allowing yourself to stay stuck in the past and you are not just focused on the future. There are people who are so stuck in the past that they are not living up to their potential, if you do this you will never grow as a person.

As for the future, it is important to set goals which you want to create and build, but don't plan every little detail in your life.

When you are living in the moment everything seems to all work out, as it is suppose to. You will be able to make decisions based on that present moment and not on past experiences. You will make clearer decisions that will be the right choices for you.

Love Yourself

It is so important to continually fill yourself up with love, respect, kindness, support, happiness, self-esteem and forgiveness. By doing this you will be your own support system. When you fill yourself up with goodness you can give and share these best qualities of yourself with others. You will be amazed at the support you will receive in return and the richness it

Always remember, you are absolutely AMAZING! Create yourself and the life you have always dreamed of. Let your true beauty and greatness shine!

Karen Gallagher

I'm the owner of Fit 4 Her, a Sports Conditioning Specialist, Nutritionist, Published Writer, Bikini Model & BioSteel Ambassador.

Female Perseverance
by Liz Gaspari

My story is about overcoming adversity. It's not unlike the stories that thousands of other women could tell – the difference is that I refuse to buckle and always manage to bounce back! Here are my strategies to help other women do the same.

My name is Liz Gaspari. Over the last 10 years, I have helped build Gaspari Nutrition, a leading, global sports supplement company, into a 100 million dollar company. As a female in a fiercely male dominated industry, my journey toward success was and is no easy feat.

Just over a year ago, I filed for divorce. The last 365 plus days have been the most challenging time of my life. During this time, I've been served with a reality check and it's surely tested my perseverance and has developed my fortitude.

Imagine being in a career, where your business partner is considered an industry icon and whose face and name are on every product you've mutually created together. The other business partner is behind the scenes, building business relationships and creating new business for the company. Now imagine that team falling apart. The business partner who's been working behind the scenes now must make their voice heard and it's a voice, that up until now, has been quietly been keeping her now to the grindstone.

Branching out on my own is perhaps the second most difficult challenge I've experienced. Remember, I work in a male dominated industry and I'm a female who's been marked as a threat to other industry people. My job now, is to show these people that I am a major reason for my past businesses success and I am a major force to be reckoned with. To date, people are finally beginning to recognize all the good I've done and all the ways that I've helped turn a garage based business into a leading global brand. It's been my ability to bounce back from adversity and to break free of the restraints that have attempted to hold me down. It's time for this woman to make her voice heard!

This chapter is about developing the part of you that's engineered to exceed and excel. Very few people learn to tap into this innate birthright, or "will power." Those that do claim two very important things:

True perseverance stems from unrestrained and pure commitment.

Once committed, something "magical" or "spiritual" ensues.

This quote from Goethe sums it up quite nicely. First, we'll dissect this quote in relation to a "Never Quit" mindset (I'm going to bold the really telling parts), and then we'll talk about ways that my fellow fems can learn to develop it. While this is a rather touchy and subjective topic, there are some things you can do right now to drastically change your life.

"Until one is committed, there is hesitancy, the chance to draw back. Concerning all acts of initiative (and creation), there is one elementary truth the ignorance of which kills countless ideas and splendid plans: that the moment one definitely commits oneself, then Providence moves too. All sorts of things occur to help one that would never otherwise have occurred. A whole stream of events issues from the decision, raising in one's favor all manner of unforeseen incidents and meetings and material assistance, which no *man could have dreamed would have come *his way. Whatever you can do, or dream you can do, begin it. Boldness has genius, power, and magic in it. Begin it now." *woman *her

Begin it now. How simple, right? Just make a choice and get started. It sounds that easy, but apparently it's like climbing a mountain for 95% of the human population.

What Goethe is talking about in that quote isn't something that one person can adequately explain to another through words alone. Unfortunately, you have to experience the truth before you can truly understand it. The good news is that once you realize the "universe" is simply waiting for your (genuine) choices, you begin to choose differently.

3 Ways to Recognize Pure Commitment

What is commitment? How do you know when you've committed to something and devoted yourself to it to the point where "providence moves too"? Here are 3 telltale signs to watch out for.

Your thinking reorganizes itself to where there is no such thing as doubt or hesitancy anymore concerning your choice. Come hell or high water, nothing can stand in your way. In fact, there are no such things as obstacles to the committed person. They are but stepping stones.

Your verbiage and vernacular changes as well. You do not speak in ways or say things that are contrary to your decision. You do not disempower yourself. You safeguard what comes out of your mouth, lest it sabotage your intentions. You begin speaking the so-called "language of success."

Rather than being an obsession, it's more of a calling. In a general sense the commitment in marriage isn't about obsession, is it?

So, basically once you stop beating around the proverbial bush of your life, coasting along or making excuses and blaming anything other than yourself…you have little else to do but commit and once you do perseverance is merely background music. It's a part of the show. It's granted.

A Fit Example

How many people say they want to look a certain way, but never do? The majority by far and then some. How many people never really make the commitment it takes to reach full physical potential, or push themselves to their personal limits or attain incredible levels of lean mass and body fat? A minuscule portion.

Why? When it can be so easy to commit. The #1 shenanigan that stands in our way is the amount of potential things to choose from. There are so many distractions literally bombarding us that it's 100 times easier to skate along being mediocre and uncommitted like most everybody else in almost every gym across the land.

- There's always time to workout.
- There's always something you can do to exercise.
- There's really no viable excuse for eating terrible food.
- Acquiring a stunning physique is but child's play to those that develop committed minds like steel traps. High fitness becomes utility to experience a fuller more vibrant and exploratory life.

The Example of Business

Here we are in one of the worst global financial meltdowns in modern history and yet, if you're broke and busted it's your fault. Flat out. Deal with it. Swallow the bitter illusions and wake up to the reality of your situation here on this planet floating through potentially infinite space.

Today there are almost countless ways to make a buck, but nearly the entire conventional system is geared to herd the masses into debt slavery (which they willingly accept at every turn) and the polar opposite of financial freedom. It's profitable!

- There's always a way to better your financial situation.
- There's always an opportunity waiting to be seized.
- No one is too good to work, especially when they're down and out.

- There's no one to blame for our lot in life but ourselves.
- There's a giant difference between a temporary want, and a long term lifestyle-type need.

Even if it were someone else's fault, to not take personal responsibility is synonymous with exacerbating the problem and further disempowering ourselves.

6 Step to a Solid "No Quit" Attitude

With that let's get down to brass tacks and discuss the 6 steps you can start to take directly after reading this chapter. If you commit there is literally a 100%, yes 100% chance that you will completely change your life. Stopping racing to the bottom to force yourself into a choice. Skip the nonsense, choose something worthwhile, commit and thrive.

Step 1: Choose and Harness the Power of Commitment

Choose. And, you likely know exactly what it is you should choose. It's that thing you have been putting off. That thing you love but choose not to invest in. That thing you are both passionate and hesitant about.

Look first to your fears. What are you afraid of? Oftentimes it is that which we fear most which possesses the most potential.

The more your choice is of service to the world, the more you will be rewarded. In fact, commit first to being of service to the world, in the best way you are capable of, and then watch as things begin to fall into place.

Step 2: Strap in for the Long Haul

As… "A whole stream of events issues from the decision, raising in one's favor all manner of unforeseen incidents and meetings and material assistance, which no man could have dreamed would have come his way" begins to emerge and transform your daily life, realize that this

isn't temporary.
- Nothing worth committing to produces short term results.
- Nothing that challenges our personal notions of "I'll never quit" has to do with temporary and superficial objectives.
- You're in this for the long haul...for the rest of your natural life.

Step 3: Capitalize on the Influence of Affirmations

Affirmations are probably the most efficient way to begin restructuring your internal monologue. They will speed you on your way to speaking the language of success. Here are some of the most popular ones you'll find after a basic Google search.
- Everything I do brings me closer to my goals.
- Everything that happens to me makes me more successful in life.
- Everyday I'm giving chance to be of service to the world.
- I'm of great value to this world.
- I refuse to quit and always bounce back.

The list could go on and on. Ideally just personalize 5 of them, and then along with Goethe's quote, repeat them until they become engrained in your psyche.

Step 4: Choose What You Attend to Wisely

Be mindful of the things you choose to pay attention to. An easy example is being sucked into the "bad news" culture of today. Just because you choose not to focus on negative things doesn't mean you don't care about them.

The biggest differences we can make in this world are within reach right now this very second. Not entangled in huge geo-political or sociocultural dramas.

The more you focus on what makes you a better person, the more value you can bring into the world. Start with changing yourself first, rather than obsessing over things you have almost zero control of.

Step 5: Transcend Physical Results

Money isn't it. Sex isn't it. Power isn't it. Fame isn't it. So, what is it then? Accomplishment? Collecting accolades? Filling a trophy case? Most often when you dig deep down into the soul of a high performer, or truly committed and exceptional person, you find that in their own minds their lives are a conversation with the universe, or perhaps a God.

The best way to get rich is in a way you don't see coming, plan for or expect. Typically these ways are discovered while doing the thing we love most; those things that bring joy into our lives and the lives of others.

The best thing to become famous for is servitude. We don't need to get pious here. What makes any business succeed or fail? The level of product and customer service.

Whatever avenue you commit to, what path you choose never to quit, make sure it is a noble and righteous path. It has nothing to do with morality, or ethics, and more to do with elementary reasoning.

Step 6: Study Great Individuals with Deep Perseverance

When you've got some time to kill, study other high achievers and let their likeness rub off on you. Search for impressions they can leave. If you're a loner, or aren't currently well-connected then fill your mental rooms with amazing people and study them as much as you can.

It's not about envy or worship, and more about learning the objective truths that drive small portions of our kind to extreme heights of accomplishment.

Outwardly and inwardly, we become the company we keep.

Here's to the bounce in each every step you take!

Liz Gaspari

I've been entrenched in the nutritional supplement industry for over fifteen years and my success has made me into one of the most powerful and influential people in the sports nutrition industry.

Never Give Up
by Nikki Giavasis

Each of us has tapped into an inner reservoir of power which we may not have known even existed until the time when we needed an exponential strength source to make it through a seemingly insurmountable situation. For each of us it has come at a time when we least expected it because that's the funny way life works. It serves up dishes of hardship and difficulty at the least opportune time because the truth is, there is no good time to go through a bad time. We look at others and we assume that they must never experience any trying times. We conclude that we are the only ones who have faced such hardships and we feel a sense of loneliness and gloom. We feel isolated and often it feels like some people got a portion of the good luck cards when we picked the joker from the deck. Eventually, whether the source of inner power we tapped into was a one time feat which got us through an enormous tragedy or it was a steady stream of strength which enabled us to keep going through times which were tough for much longer than we expected, we realize that we became better people as we overcame and persevered.

It's easy for people to look from the outside and assume the people we may admire or simply feel they got served a better or easier hand in life have carefree lives wherein everything goes their way but we have no idea the reality they face day in and day out. Those same people could be feeling the same tinge of jealousy and we would never know. We live in a society where we automatically say good or great when asked how we are. That has been researched to be the biggest and most often spoken lie told by people. We assume nobody wants to hear our problems or that there's something inherently wrong with us if we aren't having a perfect day and perfect life.

In this culture saturated by media and reality television, people have become consumed with thinking they must have all of the amenities which are given to reality tv stars who live scripted and produced life on television which the viewers believe is true reality and feel a sense of inadequacy for not living up to these abnormal standards of behavior. That being said, I think that the one true norm is that we all go through very hard times and we all like to keep it a secret because we don't want people to know we aren't metaphorically perfect. Keeping up with the Jones became such an epidemic that it wasn't until the depression during the Obama administration that people finally began to be real with each other and reveal that life isn't exactly what most have been trying to make it seem.

As a world community we are learning the importance of focusing on what is important and focusing less on the acquisition of material things to substantiate our own value or worth. The underlying truth is that no matter how hard things get, we can never give up. I realized the truth of this statement in many ways throughout my life so I feel I am somewhat of an expert on persevering through hard times and refusing to give up. It may seem from outer appearance that I may have an easy life but that is simply not the case. I'd like to peel back the layers to give you a glimpse into my life and background. I hope that by doing so, it will give you a new perspective and motivation to help get you through whatever hard time you may be facing or may possibly ever face so that you have the ability to tap into your inner power source and come out of the experience better than ever.

I grew up in a small town in Ohio and I was the only sister with four brothers. My father was 50 when I was born and a conservative Greek which means he felt that the best thing I could do was get married and have children. My mother was 21 years younger than him and very subservient to say the least. 3 of my brothers were older and from my parents first 2 marriages. I excelled in academics, ballet & gymnastics & I felt I had a somewhat wonderful life when I was a girl. My parents fought profusely in the evenings when they'd return home from the restaurant together. I would witness their fighting and it definitely stuck in my impressionable young brain. They sent my younger brother and I to Greece when I was 10 so they could try to salvage their marriage.

When I was in Greece I had a very strange bite while I was in the ocean. I ended up facing death at the age of 10. Up until that point I was active and healthy. They'd been trying to arrange my marriage to a young Greek doctor on the island. I was considered to be very pretty and I had a six pack of abs from my gymnastics training.

To say the least, from outer appearance, it seemed like my life was ideal. Nobody knew the backstory of how my parents fought viciously at night and all the sleepless nights I had. I remember being carried up a mountain to the church where they prayed over me. I was on the island of Kalymnos where my father's family originated from. I had a very high fever and most of the experience faded in and out as my consciousness did. I'm left with the scar on the bottom of my foot from the bite and the strength to know that I faced death and made it through alive. I felt stronger and more determined than ever when my health returned and I came back to Ohio. The sad thing is that the feeling didn't last long.

I'd always excelled immensely in school and extracurricular activities to that point. I was tested and found to have a genius IQ so I was put into a magnet school for performing arts before I'd left for Greece. I performed in ballet and theater and learned languages and computers. I studied science and my dream was to be an environmental engineer and powerful business woman. I also wanted to act, sing, dance and perform. I didn't feel like there should be limits to what we can do. My optimism suddenly changed because my older brother Eoun was killed in a car accident soon after I returned. I had gone with him that day in his jeep. He was getting married so he had an engagement party that night. He was following his fiancé home from the party and he hit a bump in the road and flew out of the car. He died and from there my family forever changed.

All of the big family gatherings changed and the happiness of life seemed to subside. I was old enough to understand death so I didn't wishfully believe one day he would come home. Soon after more tragedy struck. My oldest brother Philip shot and killed himself following Eoun's accident. He was on the phone with his fiancé and killed himself with a shotgun while in his mother's driveway. It was horrific. Bad simply went to worse and our golden family seemed to crumble quickly. My parents divorced. My grandmother died. My babysitter died of a rare disease.

Then, all of my beliefs were completely obliterated when I lost my virginity by being raped. I was with my younger brother and friend and we mistakenly got into a car with strangers. I had thought I was invincible as a young girl but I quickly realized I wasn't. I was even on my period but this did not stop the perpetrator. To make matters worse, since I'd been taught that you wait for sex until after you're married, I kept trying to make a relationship with the person who took my innocence because I believed I had to marry him. Eventually he did it again because people will be who they are. I was a 12 year old girl and he was a much older boy. I ended up in the hospital and again almost died. When I came to with tubes down my throat, I realized how close to dying I'd come. He'd left me on the side of the road and that was literally how bad I felt about myself because I'd been discarded and I was still completely torn apart from all of the tragedies that had occurred. I tapped into that inner reservoir of strength and I made it through. I'd love to tell you that it was easy sailing from there but it wasn't.

My inner reservoir of strength is vast and long lasting because I faced more hardships and I made it through. The great thing about life is that when we refuse to give up, we realize just how strong we really are. Knowing you can rely on yourself is a priceless gift because you have the gift of certainty that no matter what happens, as long as you keep going, you will make it through. No matter how tough it seems and how far away the light at the end of the tunnel is, you will make it there as long as you refuse to be defeated.

When you have that indistinguishable light within you, all you do is reach in and ignite it and you will shine brighter than ever before. No matter what transpires, the secret is that you don't let it beat you. Don't let it change you. Nothing about what you go through makes you less than anyone else. Going through hard times means that you were destined for greatness and your ability to persevere and overcome is a huge blessing.

Your story is your gift and when you pay it forward, it empowers you in ways you could never fathom until you do so. I did face death again with an accident when I was 18 and glass went into my bone. I also went through a horrible domestic violence situation, which is the most isolating situation that is completely horrendous. I got through those things including ending up homeless because of how bad things got. It was not long but the fact that I hit rock bottom and all I had was my perseverance and refusal to give up was enough. I ignited my enthusiasm for life and I made a vow to myself that I would never let anything defeat me. I pressed on and I realized that there is nothing that can defeat us as long as we refuse to acknowledge defeat as an option.

So many little petty things can get in the way of our life experience. When we realize that things people may say or think don't define us but are truly just a reflection of where they are in their life story. Let little things remain little and you focus on your bigger picture. Tap into your inner strength and power because you truly can overcome anything. You can truly achieve anything you dream as long as you believe you are capable. Nothing is too big and you deserve everything you can visualize for yourself and your family. I hope that my sharing may help motivate you and inspire you so you push past the tough times and keep going to make it to the light at the end of the tunnel. When you look back and see how far you've come, it's the greatest gift you can give yourself. You know you can go anywhere in the world and you can do anything you can put your mind to. No matter where you start, there is no limit to where you can finish so keep persevering and never give up!

Nikki Giavasis

I'm a talk show host, author of 4 books, CEO, founder of GG Magazine and Goddess Girls, actress, model, former NFL Cheerleader, mother of 2 teenagers, award winning fitness competitor, licensed therapist & marketing expert.

Stronger Than Yesterday
by Stacey Goldberg

Where do I begin? First off my name is Stacey Goldberg and this is a small part of my journey so far. I am a normal person just like everyone else. I have struggled with addiction my whole life, from food to alcohol. It took a lot for me to hit my rock bottom. Addiction is addiction whether it's food, alcohol or anything that is controlling your life.

I went through a lot on my journey and got lost along the way. I became very depressed and trapped in my body. I felt like there was a person inside struggling to get out and that I didn't belong in the body I was in. Back in 2008 I was in a horrible car accident where I flipped my SUV 3 times and was trapped inside and had to be cut out of my car with the jaws of life. I went completely uncontentious and all I remember is waking up and seeing a firefighter telling me that they were going to cut me out of my SUV. I remember telling him to just leave me, then I went uncontentious again.

The next thing I remember is being in an ambulance and the paramedic standing over me saying they had to cut my clothes off of me because half of the skin on the left side of my body was gone and I had glass stuck in the entire left side of my body. I blacked out again and woke up in a hospital bed. I asked the nurse if I could use the restroom and she told me that I had flat-lined for a minute and wasn't going anywhere. My heart actually stopped! I actually had died for a few seconds. I know God saved me for a reason at that point I wasn't sure exactly what it was.

The next day when I woke up and I knew it was time for a change in my life and that God had saved me for a reason. I went through my recovery it was long and hard and to this day I still have pieces of glass in my arm and the left side of my brain functions a little slower than the right side. Every time I see the scars on my arm from that accident it reminds me that I was saved for a reason.

After I finished going through my recovery process from my accident I turned to food for comfort. I am an emotional eater and when I get upset or sad I would turn to food for comfort. I let my weight get out of control and went up to 180lbs. It was such a terrible feeling. I was the chubby friend nothing ever fit and I hated myself. Certain people made comments calling me fluffy, telling me I could lose a few lbs. and I acted like it didn't bother me but inside it truly hurt me. People don't understand that one comment they say to someone that they will probably forget, will stick with the person they said it to forever!

The final straw that broke me was my ex's new girlfriend called me and told me oh I saw pictures of you and apparently he use to have a thing for fat girls. That hurt me so much! I acted like it didn't bother me but was dying inside. At that point I decided to stop feeling depressed and do something about it. I had tried everything to lose weight, Nutri System, Jenny Craig, Atkins basically anything that I thought would help but none of those worked for me.

Then in February 2011. I started working out daily and slowly cleaning up my diet. I followed women online and in magazines who inspired me to reach my goals. I started researching clean eating and exercising. This time I was determined! I threw away the scale and just went by how my body felt. I slowly started seeing my clothes getting bigger and I was going down sizes, still not weighing myself.

I remember one night standing in the fire station parking lot talking to my boyfriend at the time about what I wanted to do for work. I had been working in direct marketing for 10 years and was truly unhappy. I remember telling him "you know what I want to do, I want to help other people lose weight, workout and cook healthy food". His reply was "well that's great but that's not a long term goal. You can't make that into a career." Even though he said that to me I knew deep down inside that that was my passion and what I truly wanted to do. I wanted to help others who were in the same position I was in get out of it. The pain you feel inside that no one can understand unless they have been there. So I looked into personal training through AFAA & ACE and became certified. I also continued to research nutrition and clean eating.

Next I decided I wanted to compete. I knew nothing about competing but knew I wanted to do it! I looked up to all those women who inspired and helped motivate me over the years and just wanted to get up there and show others it can be done. You can go from being almost 200 lbs. to having the body you've always dreamt of, it just takes determination.

On May 12th 2012 I finally did it. I walked on stage for the first time, so nervous and scared. This had been my dream for so long and I was finally there, it was my time to shine and show the world my accomplishment. I also wanted to show everyone who was in my shoes that it could be done! I never realized how many people were in the same position I was and that there were other people out there going through the same thing. The moment they called my name to walk on stage I had tears in my eyes thinking about everyone who had supported me along my way. I was finally doing it! When I walked out onto the stage I felt like I was a different person. I knew I didn't die in that accident for a reason, I finally knew my purpose in life and it was to help others along their journey. You don't need to feel sad or depressed about your body. You have the power to change it. Sometimes you have to just hit that breaking point where you say "alright enough is enough!"

I decided to open an online Fitness and Nutrition Company called Stacey Goldberg Fitness & Nutrition where I help PEOPLE with meal planning and workouts. So that I can help others reach their goals. It is possible. Even if I have helped one person along their journey that is enough for me. I understand how hard it is and how trapped you feel, but I promise you it gets better! If you need anything or would like meal or workout plans please visit my page below for more information on how to get in touch.

Well so far that's just a small part of my story. I have a lot more to share with you all. But please feel free to contact me if you have any questions or need advice for personal training and help with meal planning.

Stacey Goldberg

I'm a certified personal trainer who went from 180 lbs. to 120 lbs.

How To Turn a Setback Into a Comeback
by Ryall Graber

Winning international Fitness competitions, hopping around the globe competing on the IFBB Professional Fitness circuit with an incredible group of inspirational women, being published in top fitness magazines, signing endorsement contracts, a Nutrition and Fitness consulting company that I had built from the ground up had a long string of clients waiting to sign up and I called the island paradise of Barbados home. In the spring of 2013 it appeared that I was on the top of the world.

Best friend. Husband. Checked out. Separation. Heartbreak. Divorce. Disillusionment.

Over a period of 3 months my life was falling apart at the seams. It was toxic, painful and I was living what felt like sheer hell.

So my divorce was being finalized before I could blink and I was all on my own. I wanted to get back on track and refocus but it was the most difficult thing I have ever had to do. Anyone who has had a major setback in her life knows this feeling all too well. On one level there's the desire to get moving again but on the other level, there's a deeper, more hidden craving. I wanted to stop feeling the pain. I wanted to forget this happened. I wanted my heart to stop hurting. This was emotionally ultra-tender territory. I knew I wanted a comeback but I was still drained and haunted by emotions, questions and blame.

I think we are all programmed to believe that tough times aren't the best moments to jump right into new flurries of activity. Awareness, intention, creativity and just not having hourly meltdowns are the energies required just to get through your day. But I wanted so desperately to be focused on something positive in this time of darkness in my life. I wanted to feel momentum and see light.

Do I hang up my hat and give up on my goals because of this massive unforeseen loss? How could I? Health and fitness has given me a sense of identity, become my passion, my career and a positive way to motivate and inspire others. Fitness isn't my job; it's who I am. So in the lowest point in my life I made the decision to recommit to competition and then immediately began my comeback! Over a period of 6 weeks time, smack in the middle of this emotional turmoil, I signed contracts and competed in three International Fitness competitions. And the results were beyond amazing. I claimed a second place and two wins.

Not only were these my first ever career wins but I now held the 2013 Arnold Classic South American Fitness Champion and the 2013 Toronto Pro Fitness title. This time in my life was full of the most powerful, most valuable, life-changing moments I have ever experienced in my life.

Here are my ten steps to help YOU turn your moments of sadness and into times of triumph. My steps all include the mind, the body, the heart and the spirit, as all of these elements are significant energies for your comeback.

1. Kick your 'Old Self' to the curb

Sometimes during setbacks, we just want things to be the way they used to be. We think we want our 'Old Self' back. But remember your "Old Self" was the self that was living so unconsciously that this situation was created in order to wake her up! You really don't want your "Old Self." You want EXACTLY who you are now. Bruises, disillusionment, and all. These things all create wisdom. You aren't going to be just a 'New Self'. You'll be a 'Wiser Self'. She is there, waiting for this stuff to fall away so she can rise up. So embrace the new and improved you!

2. Repressing Emotions Keeps You Stuck

Even when the worst is over, the nature of emotion is that it can creep up and take over at unexpected, and often at the times when you least expect it. Bitterness, shame, regret, anger... All of it is a part of the human buffet of emotional ranges in painful situations. There will be emotional moments; lot's of them. It doesn't mean that you're doomed to be a drama-queen forever. It simply means that there's still stuff to deal with; which is normal and totally okay.

Now you shouldn't let these emotions and thoughts rule your life from here on out however if you try to push them down, then the creative and positive energy that is meant to propel your life forward is actually working so hard at repressing these emotions that its ability to help you heal is diminished. You only have so much energy at the end of the day so give yourself space to grieve and feel the loss and sadness when you need to.

If you give them space and let them move through you, you might be surprised to find they move pretty quickly. But if you try to stuff them down they'll probably stick around and will likely cause you further setbacks in the future.

3. Be Creative not Re-active

When we spend any prolonged amount of time in a place of reaction, it is very easy to forget how to get back into the energy of positive activity (creativity). Reactivity is the opposite of creativity. And creativity is the energy that has the power to heal, transform, and change our bodies and our lives.

Often, when a setback seems to destroy someone it wasn't because of the setback itself. It was because the person never consciously moved herself back into her creative and positive space. Sadly she just stayed stuck in the energy of reacting to her life. Don't let this be you.

One of the first places to begin your comeback must be re-introducing creativity back into your being – little by little. This might be unfamiliar territory at first and can almost feel impossible but it's imperative. Creating a goal can be a great action to get the creative process started.

4. Create a goal and lay the foundation to achieve it

Now is the time to focus on YOU and what you want to achieve in your life. This will be a positive focus and some days may be that distraction that you need to get you through. Find a specific focus, write it down (this makes it more concrete and official) and make a list highlighting exactly why you want to achieve your goal. The reasons behind your goal are a very important factor in staying motivated and achieving success. Having trouble setting a goal?

Decide on three things that you want to achieve before you die. Then work backwards listing three things you want in the next twenty years, ten years, five years, this year, this month, this week and finally, the three most important things you want to accomplish today. And from there the one thing you want to focus on achieving right now.

5. Get motivated

Motivation is the process that initiates, guides and maintains goal-oriented behaviors. Motivation is what causes us to act and you are in full control of how motivated you are. Find your focus and your reason and dial into this every day. Most people are visual so creating a storyboard or cutting out inspirational photos and quotes and placing them where you can see them is a great motivator. I like using the fridge as a board as this is a great visual reminder to avoid emotional eating. This is a collage of the goals that excite you and when you look at them everyday they will soon be yours. Positive thoughts fill your mind and shape your focus.

6. Surround yourself with enablers and kick the naysayers

Surround yourself with successful, happy, resourceful and passionate people. These people will surprise you with their devotion to you and their passion for you to achieve your dreams. Why? Because these people know and understand what setbacks are – and they know what dreams are. Having this support will be more valuable than you realize. This will help you to move from bitter to better as soon as possible and be surrounded by people that lift you up and inspire you with their strengths of overcoming their own obstacles in life. This is powerful. The incredible women I developed friendships with during this time in my life all gave me the 'girl-power' to stay focused on my dreams. Not only this but we shared in some helpful smiles and life started to become fun again.

7. Identify what is and what isn't under your control

I once heard someone say, "All you can do is all you can do. And all you can do is enough. But you better make sure you do all you can do." I love this expression. You can't control destiny or fate but you can control your actions. Make sure that you're focused on the things you CAN control and not stressing about the things you can't control. This is energy you don't have to waste right now.

8. Care less about what others think

Someone's definition of you doesn't define you. Only YOU define YOU. Repeat this times ten. We all need to explore the limits of our power, push our strength find something that drives us to keep going beyond the pain and the fatigue, beyond what others have identified as the edge of our abilities. This process and time is about YOU not anybody else. Put yourself first and do what makes you happy and enables to you achieve success.

9. Failure is only permanent if you quit

Winston Churchill said it best "Success is not final, failure is not fatal: it is the courage to continue that counts". Success is never permanent. After you achieve it you have to keeping working to stay successful. However setbacks aren't permanent either… unless you make them permanent by choosing to quit.

Everybody knows that there are very few things in life more frustrating than putting your all into something and failing. But there is no reason to allow that response and the pain that probably came along with it to be the final chapter in your book. Take some time to re-evaluate what happened and then move on to the next opportunity because there's something greater in store for you next.

10. New opportunities heal old wounds

I know you've heard the expression 'When one door closes another door opens'. I have lived this! And the new opportunities that you pursue will shine light on your life and help the healing process. Be sure to stay focused on the door that's opening and not the door that's closed. You must see obstacles as opportunities as the real glory is being knocked to your knees… and then coming back. Enduring setbacks while maintaining the ability to show others the way to go forward is a true test of leadership.

A comeback is all in your control. Setbacks are always temporary and letdowns are learning experiences. They may be the toughest learning experiences of your life but there is no reason for an obstacle to turn into a permanent disaster. Let them be learning experiences and grow from them. YOU have the power to turn setbacks into comebacks and true successes. Don't let ANYTHING or ANYONE stop you from achieving your dreams. Use that setback to remind yourself how much you want that goal in your life. I did and now my vision is clearer than ever before and my passion is at an all time high. Stay empowered, motivated, focused and never quit on number one – YOU.

If you think it, you can be it.

Ryall Graber

I'm a Barbados based IFBB Pro Fitness Athlete, 2013 Arnold Classic South American Fitness Champion, Performance Nutritionist and Trainer, a Lifestyle Coach, Published fitness model, speaker, writer and the founder of RyallFitness International.

Why Didn't I Die?
by Danny-J Johnson

Have you ever been asked the question: "If you had a superpower, what would it be?"

My answer was always, to fly.

I have never wanted to become a pilot; no, that's not the flying I wanted to do. I wanted to be Peter Pan! I wanted to fly around at night and flip and twirl and sail through the air!

In 2003, I came as close to flying as one could possibly get: I became an acrobat. Talk about a rush! I was able to launch myself over 30 feet in the air from a giant swing set and do double and triple flips and land in water! The best part of it was: I got paid for it!

I was living on a high everyday and loving every minute of my life. How did I get so lucky? This is what I want to be doing forever!

Then, on June 30th, I woke up, fell out of bed and suddenly had excruciating pain running down my legs and I could barely move them… by the end of the next day, I couldn't walk at all. I was paralyzed.

After a few days in the hospital, which were a complete blur, I found out that I had a bacterial infection in my blood that was cutting off the nerve communication with my legs and almost took my life.

The doctor came in and told me I would not be returning to work. I said, "No, I need to get out of here, I will be going back on Saturday". To which she replied, "You will never be going back again. We aren't even sure if you will walk again".

This couldn't be. This was my life!! This was everything I dreamed of! It was magical, it was fun, it was exhilarating! You're telling me I may never walk again? No. I should have just died then. I wish this had just killed me.

If you've ever lived your whole life and trained your whole life to do something and your identity rests on what you can DO, then when that is taken from you, you are left feeling like nothing else really matters. Maybe you don't matter.

I started to feel very depressed and deeply wished that the bacterial infection had just killed me…

Why didn't I just die?

Then… There was Kellie.

Kellie was a dear friend of mine, I dare to say; I called her my sister, because her brother and I dated for 4 years and we became very close.

Just a few months prior, Kellie had been diagnosed with cancer. It was rapidly spreading from her colon, to liver, ovaries… all over. Kellie had a few surgeries; half of her liver removed, a hysterectomy, and now there were tumors all over her intestines. Her prognosis was bad.

In fact, just weeks before my hospitalization, I had chopped my hair all off, in preparation to shave it for Kellie's chemotherapy. We were going to show our support.

I got out of the hospital a month later; using a walker. I was still bitter, angry and overwhelmingly depressed about what I was now going to "be" if I couldn't walk. I spent days crying and taking more pain pills, because I hurt so bad, but also because it would help me sleep and forget. I wanted to just disappear in a morphine sleep and never wake up.

I went to live with my mother, so she could take care of me.

Kellie asked if she could come over.

I remember scooting to the door, with my walker, out of breath and hurting and sad. Kellie came inside, she looked at me with pity, and she said she felt so bad for me.

"This isn't fair! Why did this happen to you? I am so sorry."

Wait… what?!

Kellie? Feels bad… for me??

Kellie… who everyone knows is going to die?

Way to feel like shit.

To say that was the last day I felt sorry for myself would be a lie… but when Kellie left that day I cried and cried and cried. I cried for myself, some more, I cried for my friend's compassion, I cried for forgiveness because I just realized that I had been given a gift: to live.

And she didn't have that choice.

I cried because I realized that I had to make a choice to either let myself stay sick or I could choose to work with what I had left and find meaning in my life even if that meant I would never walk again.

I wanted to give up over and over and over again.

I stopped my pain medication and that was torture, but I didn't want to become dependent on it or become an addict. (Which was highly in my nature)

Every time I had the thought, "I wish I had just died, instead of having to work this hard"

I would think of Kellie.

I started to notice other handicapped people. I saw other people in wheelchairs and walkers like mine. They weren't complaining.

I realized that my "worst nightmare" of being in a walker, might be someone in a wheelchairs DREAM. I started to be thankful.

Thankful that I was alive.

Thankful that my infection was treatable.

Thankful that I could even use a walker.

I started to look at other people differently. I would look at the excuses of most people and realize that they have NOTHING to complain about. That many, many people in the world would give anything to have their "problems".

Mostly, what I learned, was that life is a gift. We are each given our own challenges and we must learn to deal with them, but there can always be something to be thankful for. I also realized, that even if I had never been able to walk again, there was still a reason to fight, to not give up on myself and that I have so much to offer this world. Sometimes we aren't quite sure what our purpose is here, but don't let the hard work stop you from doing THE work.

Never, ever, ever, ever give up.

Danny-J Johnson

I'm the creator of The Sweaty Betties: a global community of women looking to get fit and have fun. I'm a certified personal trainer and self-proclaimed Social Media Junkie who loves to help others live OUT LOUD.

Preserving Perseverance
by Karen Kennedy

"Not only so, but we also glory in our sufferings, because we know that suffering produces perseverance; perseverance, character; and character, hope." - Romans 5

The importance of understanding and embracing a spirit of perseverance has never been greater. In our fast-paced, high-tech, wired, increasingly globalized economy, competition is fiercer and the speed at which communications spread are faster than ever before. Have you ever noticed that when you start to explore an opportunity and it seems like the competition comes out of nowhere or even worse, that little resource called time is all of sudden lost? This intensified environment we live and work in has ensured that the businesses not grounded, will falter and fold more quickly and people will burnout. This is where the spirit of perseverance fits into your business and personal plan.

In our personal lives, the spirit of perseverance is the drive deep within our souls that ignites us to work harder, faster and smarter; to size up and stare down the obstacles in our way; to flip stumbling blocks over and discover the stepping stones on the other side; perseverance requires us to set our sights higher so we can reach and achieve more than we thought possible; for as long as it takes.

That's why I am excited to share with you the six critical keys of developing your spirit of perseverance. These principles will also help you develop a spirit of empowerment, optimism and effectiveness, but will show you how to transform those attitudes into actions, habits, and ultimately, a lifetime of abundance.

1. Get clear on what it is that you want.

You need to get clear on what it is that your spirit is pining for, the why behind your desire or passion. Visualize yourself meeting that person, making a presentation, winning a race, carrying the trophy, cashing the check… get the picture? Without a clear vision of the goals you wish to meet, you will not recognize progress even if it runs into you! A person with a spirit of perseverance is clear-minded about their goals, objectives and motives.

2. Dream and take action.

We all know how to dream, but as we get older we start to practice other get it done tactics which dull our ability to dream because we are so busy doing. The spirit of perseverance requires you to stop, reflect and dream yourself back on track, this little change coupled with taking action enables you to transform your dreams into desires, your desires into intentions, your intentions into action. The combination of dreaming big and taking action is the foundation of a life to the fullest which re-energizes the spirit of perseverance.

3. Invest and reinvest in H.O.P.E.

The competitive advantage of broadening your knowledge base is even greater for individuals than it is for businesses. The greater your supply of knowledge, the greater the demand for you as an asset and knowledge improves your decision ability. Investing in you, is one of the best ways to challenge the status quo and increase your job security.

Here are a few strategies to help you develop an enthusiastic curiosity, and enhance your ability to put your knowledge to work!

a. Keep an eye on High-Tech innovation. The spirit of perseverance needs communicative and tested tools to increase efficiency.

Having a smartphone or competitive intelligence resource to draw from allows you to remain forward-looking, for new opportunities, new tools and new ventures. As a result, you should always be on the lookout for high-tech tools, companies and people that perform at an optimal standard to drive you or your company to effectively communicate with others while leveraging tools that enable you or your company to improve and innovate.

b. Open your eyes. Often, igniting your curiosity and expanding your knowledge base can be as simple as picking up an unusual book to read. Many of the most successful and profitable ideas have come from linking seemingly unrelated ideas together – a process made possible only by a broad knowledge base.

Making time for regular reading of a wide variety of books keeps you intellectually alert, curious and creative. And broadening your knowledge base ensures that the flow of ideas, so necessary to spur the spirit of perseverance.

c. Play the field – know your competition. Research and watch your competition – their strengths, weaknesses, tactics and goals. The more you know about what other great people do right – and wrong – the better, and quicker, you are able to respond and adjust to keep going even when they pause.

The spirit of perseverance drives you to your best you and your companies unique strategies so knowing your competition means that you are always informed, but never obsessed.

d. Engage and Win. The art of active listening is a fundamental skill that few have fully mastered – despite the fact that the rewards of doing so are enormous! You can pick up invaluable information through the practice of active listening and make others around you feel a real connection as you learn by listening to them and seeking to understand –

this is the quickest way to information that is inaccessible any other way.

4. Set Standards without Compromise.

To truly strive for absolute excellence the spirit of perseverance sets a standard beyond the competition. Taking thought and actions captive, you can best sort wise risks from unnecessary ones, and having made a decision, take action, fearlessly. The perseverance persona does not gauge progress by how well others are doing, but how well they are doing. The spirit of perseverance vigorously and rigorously pursues constant improvement. It will not be detoured by variable comparisons to the other competitor. It aims no lower than perfection, and attains nothing less than excellence.

5. Maximize Adaptability and Creativity.

Many business experts believe that adaptability has eclipsed strategic planning as the key measure of a company's long-term ability to persevere. Indeed, it has become a new way to compete in a world market that is constantly changing in large-scale and unexpected ways. Improvement alone is not enough; creativity is essential. In your personal life and professional career, creativity fuels breakthroughs and personal bests.

Adopting a mindset that's akin to differentiating, seemingly wacky possibilities ensures that there is a solid foundation for breakthrough ideas to take root. Adopt the mindset that the run begins long before the race and every time you compete you will confront opposition, obstacles, challenges and pitfalls. You have the power to turn stumbling blocks into stepping-stones. It has been said that adversity causes some men to break, and other to break records. The spirit of perseverance looks for the lesson in every opportunity, and uses that information to leap over hurdles and break out of the pack. When confronted correctly, setbacks can have enormous educational benefits. They test us, challenge us and teach us, leaving us more experienced, more shrewd, more wise and more competitive.

6. Never Give Up.

Persistence is the measure of the length you will go to succeed. There is an old Buddhist proverb that states, "If you are facing in the right direction, all you need to do is keep walking." The spirit of perseverance reflects and gives light to the little actions one takes, to keep walking in the direction to your destination.

Karen Kennedy

I'm a fearlessly committed fearless fashion and fitness model, here to inspire others to seek and be their best yet!

Dream Weaver
by Sharzad Kiadeh

When I graduated from UCLA I had no idea what I wanted to be when I grew up. All I knew was that I wanted to live in LA and do something fun. I also knew that my parents weren't going to help me financially so the "something fun" I wanted to do better make me some money. LA isn't exactly a cheap place to live.

So began the struggle of my early twenties. Doing odd jobs like working part time in a spa, teaching cardio kickboxing, being a Jack Daniels promo girl at various bars, working for a creepy doctor who wanted me to chaperone his multiple "girlfriends".

The stories go on and on. I was surviving, but I wasn't working towards a career. I had cash in my pocket, but as easily as it came; it went. One month I would be on top of the world, and the next I would be busting open my piggy bank for grocery money. I had no direction and I hated it.

Eventually I landed a job as a makeup artist, which I loved… for a while. It was still a struggle though. After a few years I felt like I was stuck in a career that I wasn't excited about. Spending 18 hours a day on set with diva celebrities was no longer appealing to me. Once again I felt like I had no vision and was unhappy. I knew I needed to figure out what my next move would be. The what and how was yet to be determined.

One thing is for certain; you can't chase your dreams until you have them clear in your mind. The more specific you are about what you want; the easier it will be to go after it.

I started dabbling in blogging. I wrote mostly about makeup and beauty related things and I loved it. I submitted articles for a variety of online publications and became hooked.

Connecting with like-minded people proved to be the creative outlet I had been longing for. After a couple months of blogging (and continuing to do makeup) I decided to launch my own blog and YouTube channel. I incorporated not only makeup and beauty, but also other things I loved like food, fitness and travel. I prayed for the day that I would have a recognizable brand, and the opportunity to work with a variety of talented people in similar industries. I had no idea what to expect, I had no clue as to the amount of work it would take, and I had no friends that were doing anything similar, no guidance whatsoever. But I loved it creating content. Slowly a new dream was forming; a dream that maybe one day I could turn this into a full time, profitable career.

After two years of complete dedication I can say that building and maintaining my brand has been the most difficult and rewarding experiences of my life thus far. There is no guidebook for how to turn your brand/blog/channel into a profitable business. Every ounce of success and every dollar I've earned has come from my vision and HUSTLING. It goes back to having a clear dream.

I want to leave you with a story about a major career milestone that occurred in March of 2013. I was asked to appear as a guest on a well-known talk show on YouTube that I had been following for months. I was going to be interviewed by one of the most successful YouTubers on the planet, and one that I was personally a huge fan of. I remember wanting to pinch myself the morning of as I was getting ready to be on the show. Everything about that day seemed surreal. Walking into the studio, meeting the host and having a killer time during the show. When we wrapped I thought to myself I wish I could come to this studio every week and do what she does - but in my own way. It was crystal clear in my mind.

Fast forward about a month later and I was telling one of my best friends that I wanted my own YouTube talk show when I got an email about an important phone call that that studio wanted to have with me. I suddenly had butterflies. Every time the studio had contacted me in the past, something wonderful came out of it. When the phone call took place I had three producers on a conference call asking me if I wanted to host a new talk show that they were re-launching. Was this really happening? I asked them several times if they were serious. I asked them if I would get paid. I asked them if we would film in the same studio. All the answers were YES of course.

Now I am happy to report that one of my job descriptions includes hosting a live weekly talk show that revolves around women and women's issues. If it weren't for all the hard work I had done up until that moment and my clear vision of what I wanted I guarantee none of this would have happened. I came to find out later that literally hundreds of "professional" hosts in Southern California had auditioned for this role - but I got it - without an audition. I got it because I was prepared, had spent two years building a credible online reputation and most importantly because I had a vision.

I truly believe there is plenty of room at the top. Everyone can make their dreams come true because everyone has a different dream and a different idea of success.

Today, as I write this I feel successful. I have everything I've ever wanted including my health, happiness, a fabulous husband, wonderful relationships and my dream job. Anything else that comes my way is icing on the cake! This is still only the beginning. I know the sky is the limit and I can't wait to see what the future holds. Until then, I'm enjoying the journey!

Sharzad Kiadeh

Host. Creator. Blogger. YouTuber. Globe Trotter. Happy. Healthy. Fun. Awesome. Luxury Travel Ambassador for Michelin Guides & Host of TMVTalk at TheMomsView.

Never Give Up
by Angelique Kronebusch

"Our greatest weakness lies in giving up. The most certain way to succeed is always to try just one more time." - Thomas A. Edison

In my early twenties I was always sick. I caught every cold and flu that went around, and I was always tired. My poor eating habits over the years was catching up to me and putting on more and more fat on my small frame. I felt depressed and miserable everyday, and I would turn to food for comfort. My relationship at the time was dragging me down and caused a lot of stress in my young age, which made things much worse. I would always think to myself, "why am I putting up with this life?"

The light bulb finally turned on in my head the day I looked at a picture of myself in a tiny yellow bikini, holding a beer can. That very moment I thought, "What am I doing to myself? I am much better than this and need to live a better life!" I couldn't believe I allowed myself to become so unhealthy and so unhappy. When you feel unhappy, life is not good anymore. When you are unhappy, it's time to change things.

I decided, while I stood there holding this picture, that I was going to change my ways. I was going to stop eating ice cream and cookies for breakfast. I was going to stop eating pizza every day and stop drinking beer 3 times per week.

I was going to stop watching hours of endless TV while eating a bag of chips. What I WAS going to do is start eating more fruit and vegetables, more protein, and start working out.

I didn't know where to begin and started buying magazines and copying the exercises in my living room using dumbbells that were sitting in my closet for years. I actually enjoyed it! I also decided I would take up jogging, and I enjoyed that too. Pretty good for a lazy girl!

When I bought my first Oxygen Women's Fitness magazine, I fell in love. I wanted to be those strong girls! I wanted to be up on stage showing off my hard work! That same week I got my very first gym membership.

It was hard being at the gym at first. I was so shy and so scared to work out in front of everyone. I didn't want to look like I had no clue what I was doing, and the ripped girls in my gym intimidated me extremely. Even though I felt this way, I didn't stop. I stayed in the women's side until I collected enough courage to start training in the big gym with all the ripped guys and girls. And you know, it wasn't that bad! I felt at home right away.

One of the best things I did in my young life was dump the negative and unsupportive people. It was hard to try to be healthy when those types of people were around. I had my fair share of setbacks with food and alcohol with past friends, but I never stopped my training at the gym. I would go regardless of weather, or if I had no ride, it didn't matter. I would go even if my training partner stood me up again, and I would go even if I was tired. I would go even though my boyfriend at the time thought it was ridiculous that a girl was lifting weights and made fun of me. I will always remember the day he laughed at me when I talked about how heavy my dumbbell chest press was. He really tried to make me feel stupid. I felt so angry, but his negative attitude pushed me even harder at the gym. Needless to say, shortly after our poisonous relationship came to an end. I was not going to miss my workouts for anything or anyone! I would not allow myself to give in to excuses, and I would not allow the negative people in my life drag me down. The gym was my time to get away and unwind. The gym was my second home.

I had three goals: get in shape, become a personal trainer and help others achieve their goals, and get on stage and compete. I finally got that chance in 2008 when I decided to sign up for the WNSO Fame West in North Vancouver, British Columbia, Canada. I decided to train for the fitness model and the bikini model category. I was so excited but so nervous! I had no idea what I was doing.

2 months later, I was at the athletes meeting freaking out. I saw all the ripped and tanned people, and I thought to myself "wow I really have no clue what I am doing." I saw one girl eating yams, and another girl holding a 4-liter bottle of water. I felt so confused. I signed up for a fitness model camp after the athletes meeting with Fatima Leite Kusch, and I was overwhelmed. Fatima was going over T-walks and poses and I felt panicked. She asked me if I was putting my tan on when I got back to my hotel room. I asked, "What tan?" I'm pretty sure she felt awful for me. My poor husband drove us around downtown Vancouver at 10pm to track down some Protan, and we were painting my skin until 1am. What an awful experience that was! We had no idea what we were doing, this stuff was getting everywhere! All over the bathroom, and all over my husband. I also got it all over the hotel sheets, not good.

Needless to say, on the day of the competition, I failed miserably. I wasn't lean enough, I didn't know how to pose, I had no stage presence, and I had the wrong kind of bikini on. Even though I failed, I was determined to learn more about competing and do better next time. I researched for 1 year before competing again. The following year I did two more Fame shows, and took 2nd place at the Fame Canadian Nationals in 2009 in a large fitness model category of 25 girls. I will always remember it. I was so happy I cried on stage. Since then I have competed 12 times with some great placings. I even made it all the way to Nationals at the Canadian Bodybuilding Federation in 2012.

I have now achieved all three of my goals and have been a trainer in Kelowna, British Columbia, Canada for the last 7 years, training people hard and guiding many women to their first competition the right way. Any woman I train will never feel lost during their competition prep.

Currently my life is filled with great people that are supportive, and have the same health and fitness goals as myself. When you have that support around, goals are so much easier to achieve and life feels amazing! The biggest support I have in my life is from my husband. He has been with me through most of this, and has supported me all the way. He has gone to every single one of my competitions, and would probably be a good judge! He has helped me with my goals and would tell me what I needed to improve on for my next competition. He was a good eye in the audience.

The point I am hoping to get across to my readers is never give up on yourself. Always believe in yourself that you can do the things that YOU want to do. You don't need others to tell you if you can or can't do something. Their opinion doesn't even matter, what matters most is what YOU think you can do. If you think you can do something, go out there and do it! Life is all about the chances you take, and you will never know what you are capable of if you don't try. Only you can do this, don't wait for someone else to do it for you because it will never happen. You are the author of YOUR own novel, be your own hero. Make your own dreams happen.

Angelique Kronebusch
I'm a published fitness model, fitness columnist and figure athlete.

Living With Epilepsy
by Jenny LaBaw

Raised in a middle class household in a rural Colorado mountain town, with two loving parents and a big brother that I idolized - I had a pretty great childhood. I attended public school, had a great group of friends and influential teachers. Most early memories I have involved some type of outdoor activity. Until dark every night, my friends and I would build dirt hills, play football in the front yard and flip flop on our trampoline. As a family we spent our vacations in the mountains hiking, fishing and camping. I participated on every youth sports team possible. Life was healthy. Life was active. Life was good. Then, out of nowhere, at the age of eight, I had my first seizure.

Initially I didn't know what it was. I was twirling around the bars on the playground at recess, like I did everyday, when all of a sudden I lost strength in my right arm and came to a crashing fall onto the gravel below. Embarrassed and a bit confused, I remember quickly jumping back on the bars like nothing had happened. I felt fine except a strange "tingling" sensation in my right arm. When that sensation didn't subside and I had a few more similar episodes as the bar mishap, it was time to mention something to my parents. Obviously concerned, we made an appointment with a doctor who referred us to another, and then another and finally after several tests, it was determined that I had epilepsy.

For the next six years of my young life, I was poked with needles, submerged in scary MRI machines and constantly wondering when the next seizure would happen. The seizures themselves and crawling through the medical maze were confusing enough but the worst part of the whole deal was the medication side effects. Epilepsy is a neurological disorder without a cure. According to the World Health Organization,

50 million people worldwide have epilepsy. Medication is how most disorders are treated, but finding the correct medication and dosage can be a battle. In six years I was constantly tinkering with dosages and with which types/combinations of medication to try and stabilize my seizures. During this time the side effects were the worst part. One made me gain a substantial amount of weight, one made me experience retching attacks, one made me have double vision, I became severely toxic on one and none of them stopped the seizure activity.

Completely emotionally and physically drained with the entire process, it was time to take more drastic measures. At the age of fourteen, with the help of my family and my medical team, we decided it was time to take me totally off of medications and try to trigger a seizure in hopes of discovering what part of my brain the electrical impulses were coming from. This meant being hospitalized and under constant supervision until a seizure occurred and they were able to capture it. They tried everything to instigate an episode. They played music, they had me exercise, they deprived me of sleep, they flashed lights at my face, they tried to put me in stressful situations... all to try and prompt what I never wanted to happen again. But nothing happened. Thirteen days into this hospital stay, I was irritable, I was exhausted and I was just ready to go home. Then, what the doctors wanted to happen happened. I remember it like it was yesterday. I was sitting in the radiology department in a blue recliner with electrodes stuck all over my head, an IV in my arm and a monitor in front of me with flashing lights and weird designs continuously running across it. I was instructed to get up and press a small button attached to a tube that was attached to my IV when I felt a seizure coming on. This was going to shoot dye into my system that would somehow highlight the spot on my brain where abnormal activity was occurring and be relayed to another monitor the radiologists and doctors were observing.

I remember sitting there for several hours with my grandmother, when she briefly left the room to go grab lunch at the cafeteria. This was the only time I was left unsupervised the entire time I'd been there. All of a sudden, it was happening. I remember feeling nervous, but excited. The sensation in my arm was intensifying so I did as I was instructed and stood up to go hit the button.

The next thing I remember, I woke up and could only see bright lights and people in blue scrubs with masks and gloves on. I was yelling my brother's name. My face hurt really bad. I didn't know where I was. I was scared. Then, my mom grabbed my hand. I was okay. From there, my family and my medical team explained to me that I had had a grand mal (or tonic-clonic) seizure – the type of seizure where an individual loses consciousness and falls to the ground shaking. They told me, I did great and I did what I was told to do. I pressed the button and they found the spot. They think my seizures come from a scar on my frontal lobe caused from having meningitis as a baby. So, mission accomplished, right? I did what I had set out to do. I had a seizure, the doctors captured it, and we had an answer. Now what?

Now, time to try a new medication. This time, they were putting me on one of the oldest meds in the book – Dilantin. Nervous as to what side effects I was going to experience this time, I reluctantly started another journey with yet another medication. Much to my surprise, I felt good and my seizures were under control. Things kept getting better the longer I was on Dilantin as far as number of episodes. It was evident that as long as I paid attention to what I knew could stimulate a seizure and avoided those situations, I was going to be seizure free.

For the last 16, almost 17 years, I have been strictly on Dilantin. I have been able to do what I want despite having epilepsy. I've gotten my drivers license at 16-years old, I was captain of my softball and soccer teams, I graduated high school with academic honors. After high school I attended college where I was captain of my soccer and track teams. I graduated with a Bachelor of Arts degree in Physical Education, receiving academic honors as well. Post college I was hired on as a personal trainer at a fitness club and for the last 10 years have continued down that path developing myself into a strength and conditioning coach. At the age of 28, I was introduced to this thing called CrossFit. It is a type of exercise program involving high intensity, constantly varied, functional workouts. There are competitions within the CrossFit community where athletes compete to test their fitness. In 2010, I did my first competition and, much to my surprise, won. After my success, I was encouraged by coworkers and friends to train for the highest level of competition within CrossFit, called The CrossFit Games. Basically, it's the Olympics of exercise. So, for 6 months I trained the hardest I've ever trained for anything before, and earned myself a spot among "The Fittest on Earth" to contend for the title. In a 3-day span with 10 grueling workouts, I earned myself the title as the 6th Fittest Women on Earth.

Life is funny. Never, in a million years, if someone asked me where I thought I would be when I was 31-years old would I say a Professional Level Athlete. I thought I would have been married, with kids and living the "American Dream". Instead, I am lucky to get to spend most of my days with the man I love and have two yellow Labrador retrievers that are my pride and joy. I am living my life everyday with passion for and the ability to help others be better than they were the day before. I have a platform in this ever-growing world called CrossFit where I am able to share what I have just shared with you all. I get to educate people on what epilepsy is. Inspire people that despite adversities we are all handed, there is always a light at the end of the tunnel and positive things to focus on. So I guess, no, I am not living the "American Dream" - I am living my dream.

Epilepsy is a part of my life; it is not my life. It doesn't define me. It doesn't restrict me. It has made parts of my life hard, but it has made and continues to make me a stronger person than I would be without it.

Jenny LaBaw
I'm an elite CrossFit athlete, living with epilepsy.

Persistence & Hard Work Always Pays Off
by Tammy & Lyssie Lakatos

When we were seven years old, our four closest friends played soccer. They had practice three times a week, and games on the weekends, and every Monday morning they came to school in good spirits, recapping the highlights from the weekend games. There was nothing more that we wanted to do than to join them and play soccer too. There was something about soccer in particular that really appealed to us and that our energetic little bodies found to be so much fun. Plus, we wanted to be part of the action, the Monday chat, the weekday practices, the weekend games and after-game pizza parties, and more than anything we wanted to be a part of the camaraderie.

But this wasn't an option for us—the problem was that soccer was so popular and competitive in our town that there were never two open spots on the same team. And our Mom didn't want to put us on two separate teams and have to shuttle us to different practices and games (and now as a Mom of twins myself, I absolutely don't blame her!). Not to mention, she didn't want our teams to have to play against each other either. After, all, which team's sidelines would she sit on?!

It wasn't until we were eleven years old that two spots on the same team finally became available. We had waited so long that when the day came we could barely contain ourselves. By this time most of our friends had been mastering the craft and enjoying playing the game on a team since they were five years old, and we had waited six long years for this moment. However, when we put on our shin guards and headed on the field for our first practice, reality set in. We were bad. And not just bad. We were really bad. In fact, we were the worst players on the field, and it didn't feel good. No one wanted to pass us the ball. We didn't have any natural ability. Not one bit.

Discouraged and upset after practice, we came home to tell our parents what had happened. We shared our disappointment - and let them know that we were afraid that our teammates wouldn't want us on their team, that we'd never be as good as our friends, and we'd always feel left out of the sport that we loved. They gave us a pep talk and encouraged us to keep trying our best. They promised us that hard work and persistence always pays off and they assured us that with practice we'd improve.

The next day after school it was raining, and soccer practice was cancelled, but we headed out to our back yard to practice. We played outside in the pouring rain until our Mom made us come in for dinner and told us it was too dark to be out. Each day that we didn't have our team soccer practice, we practiced on our own and on weekends whether we had a game or not, we got up early to practice. We truly enjoyed the sport and were determined to improve - and our parents' words of encouragement, promising us that practicing and working hard pays off stuck with us.

We kept at it. Although our progress was slow, we progressively saw improvement. Initially coaches didn't play us much in games. But gradually they started to play us more and one coach in particular, began rewarding our hard work. He acknowledged his appreciation of the effort we put in at practice and the fact that we always showed up and gave 100% effort. Although we were quite far from being the best players, he rewarded our hard work by playing us more in games, even more than some good players who didn't give the effort that we displayed. Getting to play more in games was just the encouragement we needed. We really started to improve from the game-time competition, loved the sport more than ever and this all motivated us and fueled our passion even more.

As the seasons advanced, with hard work and determination we continued to improve, and we enjoyed the process of getting better. We dreamed of making the competitive high school team. When other kids were sleeping in, sitting in the air conditioning, or sitting by the pool over the summertime before high school began, we woke up early every morning to practice.

And guess what? Our parents were right! We made the team! It was one of our most profound accomplishments. It taught us not to give up and that we could accomplish anything we set our minds to as long as we were persistent and worked hard. It taught us to believe in ourselves. And it set the stage for how we live our lives.

Nothing in our business has ever come easy. Nothing. We've worked long and hard for every little bit of success. And we never give up. When times get tough we remind ourselves of what our parents taught us and how hard we worked. We think of the amazing feeling we had when we made the high school soccer team - and then we work even harder.

And we live our lives according these words:

Don't give up. Believe in yourself. Stay positive.

Tammy & Lyssie Lakatos
We are Registered Dietitians, Personal Trainers, Weight Loss Authors, Media Go-To's, Nutrition Experts and... Twins!

Healthy Mind, Healthy Body
by Agostina Laneri

The past three months have been a real emotional roller coaster for me. You would think that would make you skinny since you're sick and stressed all the time, and eating becomes less important. Not so much. When you don't eat your metabolism slows down, your body thinks that you are going into starvation, tries to hold on to the fact that it has, and stores it for the rainy days. Your body has no fuel, you become lethargic, your workouts start to suffer and you slowly begin to break down. That is what started happening to me. People think that as a trainer we have our act together and never make mistakes. I caught myself slipping. I felt bad about my body but didn't do anything, just kept going. I refused to accept that I needed a break and things went downhill, and I quickly started losing control. I started questioning myself, over thinking, overdoing and just all around making it a lot worse. But hey, I'm only human. It took me awhile to finally realize that I was no longer in the driver's seat, just the passenger tagging along for the ride. I knew I had to somehow reclaim the wheel.

But instead of letting this break me, I used it to make me stronger. It was time to regroup, dig deep inside my soul, body and emotions, and spend some time with God. Faith is very important to me. When they tell you it's a mind-body connection, let me tell you, it is true. If your mind and soul are not right and in harmony, neither will your body. Let me share something with you that helped me a lot. I love Deepak Chopra's writings and meditations, and he has seven great tips for creating this harmony and cultivating balance:

1. Take time each day to quiet your mind and meditate. That's your own special time. It can be as little as five minutes, but make time. Here's

one I use when I'm short on time. It's simple, effective and anyone can learn it. It's great for developing focus, which you can use in everyday life.

Choose a place where you won't be disturbed. Sit in a chair or on the floor, using blankets and pillows to make yourself as comfortable as possible.

Close your eyes and for a few minutes and take a few moments to observe the inflow and outflow of your breath.

Now take a slow, deep breath through your nose, while thinking or silently repeating the word So.

Then slowly exhale through your nose while silently repeating the word Hum.

Continue to allow your breath to flow easily, silently repeating So . . . Hum . . . with each inflow and outflow of the breath. Whenever your attention drifts to thoughts in your mind, sounds in the environment, or sensations in your body, gently return to your breath, silently repeating So . . . Hum.

Whenever your attention drifts to thoughts in your mind, sounds in your environment, or sensations in your body, gently return to your breath, silently repeating, So . . . Hum.

Never rush to or from meditation. Just allow the peace and calm to soak into your body, and you will carry a little bit of this peace and calm with you as you move into the activities of your day.

2. Each day eat a healthy diet. That goes without saying. A Big Mac will not make your body happy, trust me.

3. Move your body: Engage in daily exercise. Again, no brainer. Who wouldn't want a natural hit of endorphins, free of charge?

4. Take time for restful sleep. We've gotten so used to short nights with no real deep sleep. You deprive your body from some much-needed recovery. Be sure to get your eight hours of sleep.

5. Release emotional toxins. You can do this during your meditation. Holding on to negative feelings will just wear you down. It's not worth it.

6. Cultivate loving relationships. Surround yourself with people who make you feel good.

7. Enjoy a good belly laugh at least once a day. Laughter truly is the best medicine. Why not stack up on it?

Had I let life get in my way I never would've gotten to where I am today. I am now able to coach my clients through their struggles. It's not always easy to be vulnerable, but how can I expect them to trust and open up to me if I don't return it? Admitting that you're human, however simple it may seem, could be one of the hardest things. When you're feeling down or lethargic, take a moment, close your eyes, go within and find that inner fighter. Just remember the old adage: healthy mind, healthy body. The choice is yours.

Agostina Laneri

I'm one of Hollywood's most sought after health and wellness experts. I build unique relationships with my clients in order to individualize their health/fitness program.

Real Talk Real Women

Clean & Bright Perspective
by Theresa Jenn Lopetrone

"Better keep yourself clean and bright. You are the window through which you must see the world." - George Bernard Shaw

My windows weren't always clean and bright; they were dirty and foggy for years. It wasn't until I cleaned up my body that my mind became 'clean and bright'. For years I tried diet after diet in pursuit of becoming 'skinny'. Unfortunately my pursuit of losing weight never got me far. Once I lost my 5-10LBS I would go right back to my old ways of eating and socially drinking. As a result of not making a lifestyle change I would gain back the weight and a side effect of regaining this weight was feeling insecure again. My heart would race when entering a room full of strangers and even shopping in the mall alone would make me feel anxious. I remember feeling uncomfortable in my own skin and no amount of make-up, hair spray, or new clothes could change this.

I needed to hit rock bottom before I could decide to make a lifestyle change. Rock bottom happened in 2004 and this is when I gained 40 LBS in less than a handful of months. I gave up on fighting my addiction to food and just threw in the towel. Life was too stressful and if there was anything that I could rely on to help everything get better, it was food. I experienced months and months of self-sabotage. This vicious cycle would begin with eating, then feeling better to feeling uncomfortable, upset, disappointed, helpless, and hopeless and back to feeling good again each time I gave into eating copious amounts of food. Something needed to change and I knew this but I knew I couldn't do it alone. My change happened when I moved away from Canada to South East Asia. With the main motivation and encouragement of my boyfriend (now husband) I was able to create small habits of eating right, eating often, and exercising. The more I practiced these habits the better I felt and the better I felt the more 'clean and bright' my mind became. This is when I became present.

It may seem strange that all my years previous to this I wasn't living life in the present but I wasn't. I was living my life in the past and the past is what determined my future actions, thoughts, and behaviours. My perspective on life was negative; I always assumed the worst in every situation and I often over-reacted in most situations. But what I noticed when I started to become a healthier version of myself was a domino effect occurred with my mind. My body and mind were experiencing a direct correlation with one another. In other words, the healthier and more fit I became, the better my body looked but more importantly the better I felt. The better I felt the more clear my mind became, the more present I was, and the more positive my thoughts and perspectives became.

The moral of my story is that until you clean up your insides you can not clean up your outsides. When you are in a position of carrying toxins in your body you will also be in a position of carrying toxins in your mind. When you are full of toxins you will act, think, and behave in toxic ways with or without your consent. When you put toxins out into the world they are bound to come back to you which will only make you more bitter and negative. Just as Ian Maclaren says "Be kind, for everyone you meet is fighting a hard battle."

Almost 10 years later I live my life in the present, I see the positive in every situation, I am confident, happy, secure, and most importantly healthy.

Inspire and Be Inspired,

Theresa Jenn Lopetrone
I'm a WBFF PRO, Oxygen Magazine and Fit & Firm published Fitness Model, Team Blessed Bodies competitor & client support, Eat Clean Diet and Oxygen Magazine Ambassador.

Making Life Happen
by Amy Markham

I still remember the day my entire life changed as if it were yesterday. It was just a few days before my eighteenth birthday, a time when many teenagers are happily greeted with a newfound freedom to live life as they please. It all began when

I was only sixteen years old. I was sick, lost all of my friends and lost everything I had ever worked for in life. By seventeen, I had seen over 20 doctors, been told I had absolutely nothing wrong with me and was told I was just defiant and an attention seeker. Looking back, I don't blame them for thinking that. I was a varsity cheerleader, I was co-anchor on the morning news everyday, took college classes and I was a part of the "popular" crowd so to speak, being associated with so many clubs and activities. Because no one could see my symptoms they just thought I was fine. They thought I was just an overdramatic teenage girl whining about not wanting to go to school because of a headache. I was hurting for many years prior, my joints hurt, I was getting sick easily with colds left and right and I had migraines from hell. Having a typical American military family, naturally my parents wrote it off as "growing pains" and not drinking enough OJ, so I did my best and went on with life as usual, managing the best I could as a teenage girl and tried to just be as normal as possible to fit in back at school.

Then slowly as my junior semester went on, I found myself chronically exhausted, getting irritated and angry about everything, and unable to concentrate or even see properly. I remember thinking to myself, "What the heck is going on?" The only way I feel like I can describe it is sort of like a burning sensation in your head and joints, and feeling as if you hadn't slept for days. I remember I couldn't go to school on time. I would tell my mom I couldn't go today or I would just get myself up and out the door and then sleep in my car or a friend's car until the pain went away and I could walk. The worst part was no one believed I was hurting. If I told anyone they would just tell me to get over it, and that just because I was pretty didn't mean I could get away with skipping school. After a few weeks and slowly losing some of my friends, I began to stay at home more and more, and I was losing hope for life. SATs, Scholarships, college visits, the idea of even going to college was down the drain. My 4.0 GPA suddenly meant nothing, and I did in fact slowly lose everything. My life then, as I knew it, turned completely upside down.

Several months went by and we saw every specialist my insurance would allow. My main symptoms at the time were getting much worse to the point that the only way I could function was if I slept for 20 hours, woke up for a little time to eat, then showered and took some more painkillers and went back to sleep. When I was much younger, several years prior to getting sick, my parents had insisted that I be put on psychiatric medicines to "even out my mood." I was on quite a few pills daily for a few years, and I took several antidepressants and ADHD drugs. Personally, I just do not believe in prescribing psychiatric drugs for children and teens without several proper tests, and even then I think they are to be used as a last resort only. Regardless of how I felt about it, I was forced to take a cocktail of psychiatric drugs and put up with any side effects as long as they felt it was "working". To be honest, I have always been an independent, hard working, and driven child. I was told I acted 30 at 13, and it's funny because to this day at 22 years old, everyone still says the same. I did my best as a child to cope with what I had to. No amount of medicine can mask a bad childhood, it's just something you have to live through and cope with on your own terms in a healthy way.

Lets fast forward to December 2008, just a few days before my eighteenth birthday. I had gone through several weeks and months with no treatment, and was about as miserable as someone could be having not left my room or house for quite sometime. Although I was not allowed to be on the Internet or computer at my house, I had managed to buy a prepaid cell phone for myself with old lunch money I had saved up so I could keep in touch with my friends every now and then. Every evening if I was awake, the show House M.D came on and I would be glued to the TV watching it. I really loved the show so much because of my life long dream of becoming a doctor. I loved to sit there with a notebook and my medical books and try to solve the case before the end of the show. It was the only thing that made me feel happy, kept me going from day to day and gave me hope for the future.

I remember in particular there was one specific episode that caught my attention. It was about this young girl who ended up having a brain tumor with bizarre symptoms. It struck a chord with me as she had many of the same symptoms as I did. I wrote down the diagnosis and did some research with my books. As it turned out, the symptoms I had indicated a possible brain tumor, but I had no idea which kind. I tried my best researching on the internet with my little nokia prepaid cell phone too, and once I found out that there were several others out there like me with the same illness I was so relieved. I told my mother that I need to see my family physician immediately, and both she and my father agreed. I was one step closer to having an answer, and one step closer to gaining my life back.

I still remember the exact day. It was Dec 23, 2008, a cold and eerie Tuesday in December. December in Texas is rather boring at that time of year. Everything dries up, the trees are naked and it's just cold and boring, but typical Texas. I got ready the best I could and my mother took me to the doctor. It was by distance a rather short drive, but felt like eternity. I had my special piece of paper in my hand, and I told myself that today is the day that everything will change. We walked in and sat in the waiting room and waited for the doctor. I'm not exactly a religious person, but I was praying to whatever God that was willing to listen for a doctor to take me seriously for once and give me an answer. After twenty minutes of waiting and flipping through every magazine they had on the table I was finally called back.

The doctor's name was Dr. Charleston. I never saw him before but was told he was filling in for my usual family physician. This threw me off, as I was hoping to talk to someone who was at least up to date on my history, but I didn't have a choice. I sat down on the patient table and I gave him this paper. I still remember the look he gave me., he looked at me as if I was crazy and asked me why I think I may have this serious illness at seventeen years of age. I then showed him an old picture of me and I told him, "Look at me. Any normal seventeen year old girl would be out at prom, hanging out with friends, going to the mall, or playing with make up. I am here looking like this! I can't move, I can't fix my hair, my make up won't stay on because I'm crying in pain everyday and I just want to be normal. I am NOT a depressed girl. I want my life back." Think of a teenage girl with sunken eyes, pale skin, hollow cheeks and hair that is falling out in chunks and walking so slow and eighty year old would beat me. How could any doctor write that off as normal? The best answer I got before this visit was "Oh she's just depressed because of high school girl problems." The struggle to get an answer, a very simple answer, was an unbelievable ordeal.

Dr. Charleston then reviewed my paper and complimented me on my research and investigation I did on my own. Although I was proud of myself and elated a doctor had complimented me on my medical work, it was sad to think that no one would listen to a sick girl and she had to do it all on her own. Although he did agree that it was not a common illness and was something that had to be investigated further, we both agreed that an MRI would be the next step and he sent me to get one that day to check for any possible abnormalities in my brain.

After the MRI of my head was complete we went back to get the results. I walked in and sat down on the table and I looked at him and I said, "How big?" because I knew from the look on his face he had found something. When he showed my mother and I the digital image, you could see the tumor lit up by the contrast dye they injected into me. It was the best day of my life, and the worst. I felt bad for my mom because I think she really felt like nothing was seriously wrong, and that I was just had a weak immune system or something but I remember the look on her face too when she heard the words, "brain tumor".

No parent, child or anyone wants to hear those words being told to them by a doctor, but I did. For me, it meant my answer and since I am a problem solver, I finally felt as if I completed step one in getting my life back. Finally an official diagnosis. I also decided that as soon as I turned eighteen and was able to make my own health decisions, that I was going to take myself off of all psychiatric medicines and detoxify my body, and take charge of my own treatment and health.

We made a follow up appointment for after the holidays to discuss treatment and surgery options, as well as further testing. Three days before my eighteenth Birthday and two days before Christmas, I was told I had a brain tumor. I had no idea what I ever did to deserve an illness like that, but I told myself that this is a blessing in disguise and I WILL take my life back by full force.

Of course after several days of crying, moping around and being depressed, I tried to reach out to my friends to talk. Every single one of my friends had no interest in being there for me, and I was actually made fun of for being a "drop out", a "low life", and a "faker for attention" among other things. I had actually been to five different high schools and completed the amount of classes and hours needed for graduation in Texas so I wasn't a "drop out". I got my high school diploma like everyone else, I just lost the opportunity to walk with my class at graduation but looking back now, it doesn't matter anymore.

After further testing, we were able to figure out the size and specifics of the tumor. I actually hate the word "tumor" so I often refer to it as "the thing". We had a choice of radiation or surgery for treatment, and I declined surgery right away.

A few months later in the summer of 2009, and although I had lost a good amount of my hair, all eyebrows and eyelashes, I was finally starting to heal. I started to get better, but I did get enough thyroid problems to last me a lifetime and I was feeling fine for the most part. I also developed hypothyroidism, and having a tumor on my pituitary gland didn't exactly make matters better. I gained a lot of weight, and I shot up to almost 140lbs. I was normally 110lbs at the time, so that is a big difference when you are petite and small framed. The doctors never wanted to put me on any medicines for my thyroid because the doctor insisted the weight gain was "normal and a part of filling out as a woman". You can bet I ditched that doctor and the whole hospital system after that answer. I wasn't going to take yet another doctor doing nothing. Telling a woman it's ok to get fat when it is not normal for her is not acceptable. I am not the average sized woman so I refused to be treated as such. My health and weight are important to me, and I like to keep my body toned. Maybe statistics say it's ok to be a certain weight but statistics also show we have a growing problem with obesity! Having a tumor and being fat was a double whammy for me, and I was ready to take matters into my own hands.

By August 2009, I was able to start working a part time job at a local restaurant. I would work during the days, and then come home at night. I have to admit I went a little crazy at times. I was still living at my parents' house, I had no car and I snuck out, went to parties, and drank a little alcohol. I was finally normal, and I fit in without being or looking like the obvious sick girl and it felt liberating. I felt free as if I could do anything I wanted, within reason anyway.

After a month of frequent outings, I began to realize the kind of people I was hanging around. I was constantly around these kids who just smoke and drink all the time and party as if they are celebrating something great…yet they hadn't achieved anything in life yet. In my eyes, that was nothing to celebrate. I slowly began to detach myself from the group and spend more time alone, since I wanted more out of life. I grew up in a small town where most kids grow up, have a kid at eighteen, work at a bar, and then get married and divorced a couple of times and maybe go to community college if they are lucky. I wanted to be so much more than that and the longer I was around those people the more I began to see myself following in their footsteps.

My parent's got me a laptop for my eighteenth birthday so I was constantly on it. I think I was just so fascinated with the Internet since I was never allowed on it but I also was able to learn so much by researching. I spent my time researching all sorts of topics including work, cooking, and social media. I loved to read about nearly everything.

One night when I came home from work I was feeling as if I was at a dead end, and I sat down and felt as if something needed to change. I knew I wanted to be successful, I wanted to be a somebody, and I wanted to be something different. I still had a dream of going to college so I started to research about community colleges. I saved enough money from my job to buy a salvage title mustang, which I knew was my ticket out of that small town, using "college" as my excuse. I applied to a few colleges, was able to get accepted at one about two hours away and I packed up my car and left. My parents were against it but I knew it was the right decision for me. I needed to leave and I knew there was another world out there waiting, and I refused to settle for normal and average. I left with only $20 to my name and a dream. I didn't care what I ended up doing, I just wanted to be the best I could be and be successful. I knew if I could get this far after losing everything, I could get even farther having all the opportunities in the world and having full control over my life.

So that was it... I had my $20 in my pocket, a suitcase and a car with just enough gas to get me to where I was going, and a dream. I've always been that kind of girl, that "girl on a mission". I believe if you have a dream, you have no business sleeping and dreaming about success. You have to be awake every minute putting in hard work to bring that dream to life. I want to live my success, not see it only when I'm dreaming. My goal is to make my success real. It was never really about the money or the fame. Just making and reaching goals you set for yourself and pushing it as far as possible.

Right after I got into town, I got an apartment and started college right away. I went to school everyday, and did everything I thought I was supposed to do as a student. I remember sitting in class one day, and my teacher was asking us what our career path was. I sat there, and was confused and a little shocked by the answers. My peers replied, "Vet Tech, RN, Physical Therapist, Pharmacy Tech" and suddenly I realized that I was in the wrong room. Not that those professions are bad at all, I just didn't want to be ANY of those, and my dreams of becoming a doctor were dying the longer I was in college anyway. I realized college was not meant for me, and that no algebra or chemistry formula was going to translate into a formula for success in the real world. Maybe in pharmacy tech world, but certainly not Amy's world.

It was something that needed to be learned with real world experiences. Maybe part of my feelings stemmed from being sick and having almost lost my future completely, but I don't like to have limits, or for someone to tell me this is how much you are making per year, when you are working, and what degree I need to get a job that has little room for the growth I was seeking. I was seeking something far beyond that, something a degree would never get me. I didn't have my parents paying for my college or someone paying for an education so I decided I was going to embark on my own path. I had no idea what path I was embarking on exactly but I knew this was my last chance to make it for myself.

After I was back to being somewhat healthy, I was told I should model by a few people I knew. I met a few agents along the way, but almost every agent I met wanted me to pay for some scam modeling school, which we all know is not necessary. I decided that it was worth a shot, after all I had nothing to lose. I started from the bottom, working as a car show bikini model to get started and now I travel and get to shoot for some of the coolest magazines on the planet.

To make a long story short, here I am now almost three years later, being one of the most searched celebrity glamour models in the world and having posed for several high end magazines such Maxim, FHM, GQ, Esquire, and Vogue. It was up to me to change my life and become my own person, and carve my own path to success. I truly believe it took me losing nearly everything to get to where I am at today. Every mistake I ever made, everything I could have done better…it all had to happen exactly the way it did for me to be here where I am today. Everything you need to succeed you already have. There is no "Why me?" attitude and no giving up.

The key is to set small realistic goals and stop at nothing to reach them. I always look at my "mini goals" as steps to the ultimate goal. Just like with diagnosing myself was step 1, shooting for my first big magazine was step 1 to get to the bigger publications. If you set small goals and start accomplishing them, you will taste the sweetness of success and be hungry for more. No matter the circumstances, your career goals, your past or present, you have all the tools you need to make the first step in bettering your life.

Everything you need is within your mind and soul, and the power is within YOU.

Amy Markham
I'm an International Cover Model.

Fit Mama is Pregnant Again
by Christie Nix

I worked hard! Losing 55 pounds twice wasn't easy and I certainly didn't feel all that great about myself after my babies were born. I was left with the after affects of pregnancy and it couldn't come off fast enough. I wish I could say it was the recommended 25 pounds but with the first two it was more like 55. Having always been a fit and athletic person pregnancy was a chapter of life that was a struggle. I didn't feel good because I wasn't exercising or eating right. I didn't exercise during pregnancy because it was the only time I dealt with feeling so uncomfortable in my own skin. After each of the girls I busted my butt to lose the weight. I just wanted to feel good in my clothes again, make sure my husband had a wife he could be proud of and for me to be okay with what I saw in the mirror.

When my second daughter was 2 I took my fitness to the next level and trained for figure competitions! Of course starting at an ideal body weight was helpful but now I was in the business of making muscle. Before she was 4 I did 3 figure shows placing in two of them! I loved my strong body, my level of fitness (gym Rock star you could say), and constantly desired to get stronger, faster, all around better. I took what I knew in my head about proper nutrition and put it into practice, cleaned up my diet for life not just competing and committed to a healthy and balanced lifestyle not to be skinny again but because it's truly what I love, practice and preach to my clients.

Shortly after our youngest turned 4 my husband and I decided to go for a third. A new child to love, a new baby to hold, perhaps our first boy, so much to be joyful about, but what a SETBACK that would be. Physically a setback as my body would obviously change, my muscle mass would begin to decrease, my skin stretch again, and of course the unknowns that come during the birth process. Some would ask why you would ruin all that hard work and I couldn't argue with that question.

Not only did I acknowledge the physical setbacks but the mental struggle also. Fearful of this being the pregnancy that does me in and I can't get my body back, can I handle my passion for fitness with two busy daughters and a newborn, how will I adapt emotionally to not being the fit and fierce woman I had been the past few years.

I had come so far and I hadn't forgotten how my body handled pregnancy the first two go arounds. I wish I could say I completely embrace the beauty of pregnancy but that wouldn't be the truth. I know in my heart I'm blessed to carry a child, to have children, and what a miracle that is. But my head tells a different story.

Aware of all this, and my selfish, self absorbed thoughts God always challenges me to stop thinking about me. So last October (2012) shortly after my 31st birthday I was pregnant. Determined to not let this be a miserable pregnancy and let my selfish nature win I made a plan so this setback could be a step forward in so many ways.

So much of my training effects how I function so being a lazy preggo was not going to work this time. Regardless of how I feel I look, how I feel while I train, or how big my boobs got I made exercise a priority. I kept my usual gym time and while I didn't always feel like it went and worked out, and I worked out hard! Having been active, strong, and agile before I became pregnant continuing to train was perfectly safe for baby and myself.

Not only did I train and exercise I was mindful of my nutrition. Certainly I indulged more than I would have if I were not pregnant but keeping similar eating habits would make transitioning post delivery that much easier.

As a personal trainer I continued to work up until the last 6 weeks.

Keeping my clients focused, challenged and strong kept me even more so in the arena of fitness.

Other than my changing body and insecurities about my appearance I didn't let any of that take me out of what I know I love.

My healthy baby boy is now 4 weeks old, and of course I am in love! He is the perfect addition to our family. I am on the other side of this "setback" working to get my body back. My plan to make this life lesson a step forward proved beneficial! I still gained weight obviously but 35 pounds is way better than 55 (and all of my babies were small so that isn't a factor). My confidence during this last pregnancy was the best it had been for all three. My energy and activity level stayed high throughout the pregnancy and I was able to keep up with two busy daughters. I even coached my oldest daughter's soccer team all the way up to 8 months pregnant. My post delivery recovery was easier than expected and I was able to start light exercise just two weeks after delivery.

The post baby body is quite a change from the fit mom that stepped on stage two years ago but because I know this is my lifestyle and I maintained it as such throughout I'm hopeful to get back where I was.

Being fit before or after children is a reality, whether it's for one child or 10, you just have to make up your mind that you will do it!! I'm thankful I was able to get over myself enough to add more love and life to our family and will fight like hell to be a fit mama of three because all setbacks make for amazing comebacks!!

Hopefully you will find me on my Facebook and see the progress I've made on the journey to get my body back!!!

Christie Nix

I'm an Army wife, mother of 3, personal trainer and am passionate about training and nutrition.

Empowering Women Worldwide by Elisabeth Nuesser

I was a single mother for six years, the only sister with 6 brothers and a woman in a male dominated profession of Mixed Martial Arts I have been through many struggles in my life and I will continue to embrace many more battles to do my part in empowering women around the world.

It all started February of 2006, I had come home from a long night of bartending and waitressing I had drank too much Monster energy drink and couldn't sleep…I woke my husband Jake up and had told him about the rough night I had and was very emotional. I went on about where my and our lives were really going at that time. We had just had our son Jase together he was 4 months old and Justyne our daughter was 7 years old. I started working at a near by bar/restaurant to make extra money. I couldn't sleep that night because I was too shaky from the energy drink so I asked Jake to stay up for a bit with me, we turned on the T.V. to the Spike TV channel and started watching old re-run UFC fights (the male dominated sport of mixed martial arts) and it was that night at 3AM that I came to the realization that I really loved this sport.

I watched the fighters walk out into the cage and I noticed women in the audience cheering them on. I knew women were training in the gyms, what I didn't know until later was that there were women who were fighting too. As I watched that idea more closely, that "light bulb" went off in my head. It was that "Ah Ha" moment in my life. I loved this sport, I love watching it, but I don't want to wear designs on shirts with skulls and blood splatters on it.

I wanted to wear pink clothes cute, sexy, and tough designs to represent the sport as a female. I asked my husband (who is a graphics designer) how come there isn't anything for women to wear to support the sport? He said I don't know, no one has ever done that. I said I would wear cute gear if someone made it for girls like me. He then challenged me and said why don't you start your own clothing line? I said fine I will! That night we stayed up until 5AM coming up with different sayings for shirts, one of them is still being sold on our website www.FightChix.com "I Break Hearts and Faces" it's been the number one seller from day one. That night or should I say morning I came up with the name FIGHTCHIX the name was everything we wanted the vision to be about.

Shorty after, Jake designed the logo, which we never made any changes too. Once he showed me he had nailed it! I knew after seeing our logo that this was something that was going to be BIG! A week later he designed a website we started a Fight Chix Myspace page and we started marketing it. Hours later we were being asked to sponsor a female fighter (Michelle Waterson) I had no idea even how to do that. We came up with this idea and now how do we make this a real business. With much persistence, extreme hard work and dedication, having that entrepreneurial spirit in me many trials and errors to learn we are still trucking along. As days, weeks, and months went on and the timeless efforts we put into this company becoming what we call our "third" child has turned into the last almost 8 years has been quite a journey.

From all the Ups: Signing a licensing deal with Spencer's Gifts and being in over 400 retail locations, being nominated for Best Lifestyle Brand in 2010 for the Fighters Only Awards, sponsoring some of the best female athletes in the world including: Miesha Tate, Cat Zingano, Kelly Kobald who fought Gina Carano, Roxanne Modafferi, and many more.

Let's not forget the downs: Working at night bartending/waitressing to pay bills and cover costs on Fight Chix doing hair clients during the day to make ends meet being the best Mother I can be to our two children and wife to Jake all while doing Fight Chix full time. Jake also worked full time during the day as well, he was a bouncer on weekends for extra money and did Fight Chix designs at night, he was also laid off from his full-time job for quite some time as well during this journey. Fight Chix was an idea and a start up business. We had no idea would be so rewarding and so challenging at the same time.

We found through this entire process that the name Fight Chix wasn't just about supporting the sport of mixed martial arts for athletes and women fans, but that we had been touching lives around the world and didn't even know it. Each individual identifies themselves with our brand and logo in their own way. From Breast Cancer survivors to everyday women that wear our clothing items because it makes them feel empowered and confident, to the athletes or women that want to workout or train in our gear.

We reached out to people asking for testimonials and the response was overwhelming. We had found that women wore our clothing because it helped them overcome their own struggles in life. One woman told a story of how she was in a domestically abusive relationship and wearing our apparel reminded her that she is strong and not to have anyone put her down. Another was a woman in the military in the K-9 unit. She wore our apparel because it helped her feel confident that she could do her job overseas and being the only female in another male dominated atmosphere. The Fight Chix logo with a female silhouette with her fists up defending herself became their own symbol of empowerment. Let's not forget the men too! We have a lot of male fans as well who support our vision and female athletes. I have learned so much through this whole process and I am very grateful for the people that I have connected with and the experience of it all. Fight Chix has become a lifestyle brand and a voice for girls and women everywhere.

Miriam Khalladi

I will leave you with some advice that I hope you will take with you after reading my chapter. It is very important to Believe in your passion, go after your dreams, do what you love and love what you do. Follow that idea and intuition.

Thank you for taking the time to read my chapter and I hope that I have inspired at least one of you to go after your dreams!

Love & Light,

Elisabeth Nuesser

I'm the female CEO of Fight Chix Apparel, mother of two great kids, a wife, a hair stylist, and an entrepreneur empowering women around the world!

Finding Your Passion & Living Your Dreams
by Shannon Petralito

From a very young age we are all asked the same question, "what do you want to be when you grow up?" Children are never afraid to dream. Do you remember having these amazing ideas of what it is you wanted to contribute to the world when you "grew up?" What were you passionate about? Whatever it was I'm sure when you were younger there was not an ounce of fear in announcing it to the world. You were not afraid of being laughed at, you were not afraid of failure, in that very moment in time you were confident that you could be that something! You believed you could be whatever it is you wanted to be! You were passionate about your goals, dreams & aspirations! Do you remember lying awake at night thinking of how you could get there and what steps you needed to take to live your dream? I sure do!

Something happens however when we get older, we somehow lose that confidence and we somehow think our wildest dreams are not worthy of pursuing. These dreams seem too far-fetched and too hard to reach as we get older. Sometimes it's because our lives take us down different paths that lead us to unexpected experiences and somehow we get wrapped up in the moments and forget about what we really want out of life and what it is we really desire.

Growing up I remember wanting to be a range of things from a famous singer to a trainer at SeaWorld! I believed with all my heart I could! At one point I took voice lessons and learned my career in singing was short lived! At another point I decided to take courses in Marine Biology and Chemistry so I could work with marine mammals but soon discovered that the higher levels of math were not my strong point. I continued with the Biology courses not knowing exactly where they would fit in in my career but I stuck with them anyway and dropped the Chemistry. I tried like heck because one thing I am not is a quitter and I am not afraid to fail. I am more afraid of not trying and asking myself what if!

Years passed and I graduated only to be left continuing the job I had throughout college - working nights as a bartender. I began to wonder what is my passion? What is it I really want? What was I going to do with my life? I honestly felt empty and lost! I could not answer the very question that I was so eager to tell everyone when I was a child! What happened? Was it that I grew up and the reality of the world made my cynical?

In a panic to "find myself" I took the advice of my mother and went back to school to get my paralegal certification. Was my heart in it? No, but I felt I needed to "find my passion" by trying different things, maybe eventually I would run into something I loved? Well, it wasn't becoming a Paralegal. Back to the drawing board I went and continued with my "safety net" job of bar tending. Was I happy? No! I was depressed & miserable - I felt bad about myself. It was hard to watch all of the women my age around me with careers while I was now a new mom tending bar! It did a number on me mentally!

Alas! Then came fitness! Exercise has always been part of my daily life in one form or another. After I had my son I decided to challenge myself and compete in a Figure Competition to get in the best shape of my life and to focus on something positive to help me forget about how unhappy I was with my job. Was I nervous? Heck yeah! I had no idea what to expect. I am a thrill seeker by nature. I thrive on the rush and adrenaline! Little did I know that this random decision would change my life and ultimately help me find my passion!!! I soon discovered that working nights and getting in at 4am and up at 7AM to train and take care of an infant did not mesh well. This is where the leap of faith happened! After 15 years I decided enough was enough and I decided to go for it and give 100% effort into building a career in the fitness industry!

After all I loved working out, I loved competing, I loved soaking everything in that I could about nutrition and fitness and I really loved sharing my knowledge and passion with others! Could I have finally found my calling? I believe I have! I love what I do!

As with any business or career change it takes time to build and it takes patience in networking and making connections but if you are driven and passionate enough you will get there! Doors will continue to open and some will close presenting bigger & better opportunities. No experience is ever a bad experience, think of them all as learning experiences and opportunities for growth! I without a doubt know I have made good decisions and not so good decisions but all resulted from not being afraid to try. I know I have so much more to learn and I know that many more opportunities await but I have to be bold enough to go after them! How else can you live your dreams and find your passion? You don't just stumble upon them - you have to be courageous enough to put yourself out there and try new things!

I spent many years believing that some people have good luck and some people have bad luck. I believed that some people were just fortunate enough to have great opportunities present themselves while others like me just made the wrong decisions and that was it - I had to make the best of it. I somehow felt that if I missed out early on my calling then I was destined for whatever was coming my way - again feeling lost and angry!

It wasn't until I made this decision to take my interest in fitness to the next level that I discovered my passion and began to dream big again just like when I was a child!

I began to revisit my faith, I began to think positive and began to truly believe that if I worked hard enough I could make things happen! I began to believe that I deserve to be happy and to be successful and that God would present me with the tools I needed to get me there!

Just about five years later here we are reading a chapter in a book that I am honored to have been asked to write! I would never have imagined that I would be sitting here at my computer writing my thoughts and hope that they motivate and inspire others in some way!

After years of soul searching and many learning experiences and some let downs my path has led me to what I believe I was meant to do. I truly believe I was meant to utilize my knowledge in fitness and health to educate & inspire others. I love what I do and I am PASSIONATE about it! It is an amazing feeling to help people become more confident in themselves and begin to love themselves as they should.

I used to be that person, feeling lost, uninspired and unsure. I want to pay it forward and tell each of you that no matter how young or old, not matter how many mistakes you make there is always time to find your passion & live your dreams. Each day is a new opportunity so make the most of it! There will be bumps in the road and there will be days you feel like you're getting nowhere but as long as you keep moving forward you are getting closer to your success!

Finding your passion comes easy for some of us for others it may take a while but I really believe that no one should have to "settle" and feel that this is the best life has to offer them if they are not truly happy with where they are. Everyone deserves happiness and everyone deserves to experience something they are passionate about.

We have all heard the saying "nothing worth having comes easy" if you truly want something bad enough you are most likely going to have to work for it. I don't really believe that those who we see as "lucky" and having it easy really do - in fact, I think that the less you have to work for something the less rewarding it is and you will always in a sense feel an emptiness or a void.

If I can close this chapter with one final piece of advice it would be this: Pride and passion are found through working hard and remaining humble. Stay focused and dedicated to your goals and as you learn and succeed always be generous enough to share your experiences with others. Have faith and know that there is always a chance to find your passion! Doors open doors close but opportunities are always present you just have to be receptive to them!

Live with belief, live with faith, live with passion!

Shannon Petralito

I'm a WBFF pro figure athlete, Ms. Figure Universe 2011, CPT, fitness model, health & wellness expert. I have my own business called Shannon Petralito Fitness where I'm helping women live happier & healthier lives!

My Life is a Progression, Not Perfect
by Jessi Piha

I'm exactly where I am supposed to be.

In a city where women are dying to be, to look, to present themselves as perfect, it's a miracle I became a person I can be proud of. Trying to be perfect is magnified by being judged daily on social media - how many "likes" you get on Facebook can mean the difference between having a good day or a horrendous day. It is a delicate balance to find an inner peace amidst the choir of voices giving their feedback every second.

When the world is focused on finding people's personalities on the Internet it puts me in a vulnerable place: Do I put myself out there and risk the criticism? HELL YES!! is the answer to that question. I know that everyone has an opinion and their own way of expressing it - that's what makes this world so beautiful - we are individuals, we are all unique.

The trick is to not take it all personally. I wasn't taught that as a young girl and I wish I had had a guidebook, a 101 on how to survive in Los Angeles, but I didn't. I wish my parents hadn't divorced, I wish I had made better choices with my relationships, I wish I had never known the intense feeling of fear and anxiety that debilitated me to the point of taking drugs, drinking and isolation. I had been given material things growing up which led me to believe I was getting it all, everything I wanted, but was it everything I needed? It wasn't until I got sober that I did some deep painful and insightful soul searching.

I believe there has been a plan for me all along. In my early 20's, I was randomly (if you believe in accidents) asked to work the front desk of a health club. This became the stepping-stone that triggered my interest in fitness. Ironically, the 20 years to follow were the unhealthiest of my journey. Anyone who knows me now post-addiction can't fathom the path of destruction that led me to my present. It doesn't make sense and it shouldn't have worked but it did. Someone up there wanted me to teach this message; to have it all come to fruition in a way that could maybe reach just one person who is suffering like I did. After getting my act together I came back to the one one thing that I knew, Pilates. It grew from there to a place I never thought I was capable of: a confidence and command of my body and mind, a true work in progress every day. I get to help change lives and connect with people in a way that not many get to do.

I'm a free spirit, a hippie, "Old school," so it's difficult to hang on to that in the world the way it is now. I miss answering machines, I miss the anticipation and the waiting to come home to get messages, communication happens fast and everyone is rushing. I miss taking photos and taking the film to be developed and getting together with friends to pass photos around. I want to adapt and at the same time I resist and that takes me back to a place on anxiety I lived with for so long. So I keep on adapting and accepting and having faith that there is a safe place in my soul that is always going to be here for me and I don't have to look to the past or the outside to find it.

I'm realizing just this moment as I'm writing that surrendering and giving up are two very different acts and surrendering doesn't' mean I'm weak, it just means that it's ok to let go. I've never given up, I hate the word "can't," and as long as I always try I can be proud of myself. The first month of getting sober put me in a vulnerable position to rely not only on my own self will but also the support of total strangers. Although we were all working towards the same goal of getting clean I didn't know these people and after so many years of isolation it was terrifying to let my guard down. As it turns out that experience was one of the first of hundreds of blessings to cross my path. Of course at the time I wouldn't realize it but the parallels now concerning my career are crystal clear. The amazing compassion from people I barely knew got me back on my feet. I had to bravely commit to something so frightening in order to get the life I wanted. The life I get to experience now is a direct result of a miracle that happened to me. I pay it forward by empowering my clients to reach out, let go and jump into something that may be scary but the rewards are far greater. I'm a cheerleader and motivator in my classes but when I have an opportunity to get humble and share with them how I've had the same struggles as they are having, the same fears, it breaks the barriers even more. It makes them vulnerable and that's when they get to have THEIR breakthrough.

Being uncomfortable is a feeling that lived inside me, it was and can still be painful. It's an interesting dichotomy because learning to tolerate being uncomfortable is how I teach my fitness classes, learn to live and love the pain and the burn and you will evoke change within your body. It's impossible not to get attached when I am witnessing miracles, breakthroughs and goals being achieved. What makes me the teacher I am today is the ability to be relatable. Walk the walk, to talk the talk. The sense of empowerment I can help someone feel transcends far beyond just doing a set of push-ups or holding a plank. This year I had the privilege of working with a girl throughout her first pregnancy. Three times a week I was blessed to watch her on her path leading up to miracle of giving life, she developed a strength and a glow and I was impressed every time she just showed up for class. When that little girl was born and I got to hold her when she was 9 pounds and just 3 weeks old, was a moment that touched my heart and that feeling of happiness for someone else's joy is an unbelievable emotion.

These moments are gone in the blink of an eye. Progress is time just moving through space and the perfection is some fantasy, an end result

I have created in my head. It isn't' real, the moments are real and they are beautiful.

Jessi Piha

My journey through health & fitness has had its ebb and flow, but because of my dedication to fitness and roots to this community, I'm now blessed to be recognized as one of the top fitness teachers on the Westside.

A New Perspective; A New Stage
by Lacey Pruett

I believe life is a stage. I believe it's okay (and necessary) to take pauses and be occasionally selfish. I believe you should create your own standards and your own normal. I know that boundaries are not just healthy, they are life saving. These lessons contradict my others-centered upbringing in small-town America, being educated in Catholic schools. Furthering the contradiction, I became my own worst enemy, before I learned to be my own best friend. Learning about self-compassion allowed me to create a new normal for myself and for my family, and even better, I finally started to live life abundantly and remembered to have fun.

Being the second oldest of four daughters provided opportunities for me to stand out and be a little controlling from the beginning. When my sisters and I were home alone, we had our own stage and our imaginations went crazy. In one afternoon, we were actresses, singers, and dancers. My older sister, Bridget was the shy, reasonable one. I enjoyed taking the spotlight from her, and she didn't mind. Conversely, I learned loyalty early on as well. Let it be known that I can complain about or poke fun at my sisters - you can't. When my two little sisters joined the party, they never had a chance. I was already louder, bigger, and bossier.

In college, it got worse. I was two years into aggressive pageant training, still having not made the transition toward a more balanced perspective of true beauty and health, already having won two separate titles with Miss Texas USA pageant system. Texas Tech University in Lubbock, TX would be the stomping ground for my greatest lesson to date: Do not conform to the standards of this world, but rather be transformed by the renewing of your mind. My controlling nature fit well within the strict diet and exercise routine I followed. No, it wasn't healthy, and I was headed for death. I knew I couldn't keep going at the pace I set for myself, racing after what society demanded of me. Seeking Earthly crowns, degrees, status, and outward beauty consumed my days, when I should have been investing in my personal health, positive relationships, and defining my own standards of self-worth. I got help from a team of professionals who taught me to change my perspective a bit. We got to work on new perspectives for health, beauty, relationships, and success.

If you've ever undone relationships, you'll understand the pain that ensued after making this commitment to myself. Telling someone they no longer fit into your new world is tough. Even more difficult, is shunning the activities you used to enjoy - so you thought. Getting yourself to understand your decisions is a challenge, followed closely by the difficulty of helping others understand your decisions. Despite all of the hurt, you (your health, and your well-being) matter more. Closing my pageant career, gaining 10 pounds of muscle by setting boundaries in my exercising and nourishment, and two broken engagements were some of the first decisions made within new personal boundaries. Leaving a wake of broken plans and hearts gifted me with moments of insecurity and pain; however, I carried a peace in my heart that remained unexplainable.

My 12-year corporate career came about just as it did for most college graduates at the turn of the century. When I signed on with Southwest Airlines, I knew I was in for something special. The promise of growing with a respected company seemed like a great fit for a newly-single girl in the big city. It was only about five years into my career that I realized I was on stage again. This wasn't the pageant stage; however, titles still provided power and prestige and people everywhere were craving both. Even worse, youth and beauty were curses, and I fell right back into the quest for society approval at the risk of my own health. The long hours, demanding after-hours social life (not attending wasn't an option), and always looking ahead to the next goal instead of appreciating and celebrating existing accomplishments, led me back toward a life of unhealthy perspectives and without appropriate boundaries. The corporate stage was ruthless, even at a good company. Remember that great lesson I received in college? I fell right back into conforming to the standards of the world instead of transforming and renewing my mind. Damn it.

Despite a successful career, being financially and socially content, my spirit was unsettled and I longed to nurture something more than just my career and social life. I employed the help of two holistic wellness advisors to help me figure out why I was still fatigued and lacking fulfillment. Together we dissected my world, perspectives, standards, boundaries, and overall well-being. We had some work to do. To be honest, before this time, I never really wrote out a list of core values, or asked the questions: "What matters most to me?" or "Does my daily agenda match up with these core values?" Sifting through how I lived my days and what mattered most to me provided answers to my non-fulfillment. I learned that up until now, I've ignored two key aspects of overall wellness. My spiritual strength needed work and my perspectives relating to success, relationships, and health needed toning.

At this season of my life, I really enjoyed running as my physical and mental therapy. With each distance race I completed, I felt past insecurity and pain fall off my shoulders and started creating new perspectives for my life. There's nothing like a marathon to send you on an emotional roller coaster through your past, present, and future. With each step, I reminded myself of how blessed I was to be on a healthy journey toward my destiny. I enjoyed the fitness challenge because I was desperate to see what I was really capable of. I craved competition again, but now it was with myself. The physical challenges were great, but I really loved how strong I grew mentally and spiritually. I didn't understand, at the time, that I was being conditioned for my most challenging title yet.

I'll always be grateful to my former company for introducing me to my husband. I met him at the office, at a time I wasn't looking for a romantic relationship. I just figured out how to love myself better, and I wanted to hold onto that for a bit before adding someone else into the mix. I was genuinely fulfilled, maintaining my boundaries, and challenging myself daily with my career and some new opportunities in the health and wellness industry. I never dealt with my control issues. Crap.

If there's one thing you lose in marriage, and as part of a blended family, it's control. While I should have allowed some more preparation time for my control detox, six months into a new marriage didn't afford me that luxury. Since we're being real here, it sucked at times. It wasn't anyone's fault, really, and looking back, we all did pretty damn great with the cards we were dealt. When I saw the struggles we were having with our new roles, I offered the idea to create our own rules. Once we decided together, as a new blended family, to design and build our new normal, our new perspectives, and our new boundaries, the gloves came off... magically. I was no longer, step-mom but now bonus-mom. They were no longer my stepchildren, but rather my bonus children. We committed to appreciating our unique family structure and the opportunities we have that others might not. My husband is a daily, living reminder of maintaining healthy perspective, balance, and a constant (somewhat aggravating) reminder to have a little fun. He keeps first things first, and doesn't care whether or not you agree with what he considers a first thing. He is always grateful and always quick to count blessings. When I waiver on my own quest for this type of balance, he's my encouragement.

Losing the leadership title in corporate America was difficult, as was losing the 12-year career that created a lot of my identity. Taking the leap of faith toward working for myself was the most exciting, creepy, and peaceful leap I've taken, second only to marrying my husband and relinquishing control over aspects of my life. Once I stopped conforming to the standards of the world and focused more on transforming my mind, my world opened up. New titles of wife, bonus mom, spokesperson and advisor have fulfilled me more than I anticipated, and I've just started. As Mrs. Texas United States, I enjoyed speaking to groups of young ladies about how to properly care for themselves in a holistic way - body, mind and spirit - and that no matter their circumstances or goals, create your own standards and rulebook. Never give up on yourself. Never conform to society's standards of beauty, health, and success. Create your own normal and perform well on that stage.

Lacey Pruett

I'm a Corporate Spokesperson, TV Host, Mrs. Texas USA & Healthy Housewives Cast Member. As a former Mrs. Texas USA, I'm no stranger to the spotlight or competition & feel there's a positive way to utilize both.

I Crashed Into My New Life
by Abigail Rich

I should be dead according to my doctors. They told my family that they should donate my organs, that I wouldn't make it through the night. Well, I did make it through that night and what a wild ride my life has been since then.

Let me tell you a little about myself. I was born and raised in Dallas Texas. All through my childhood and all through school I have been a caretaker sort of person. I have always liked taking care of people. Not in a mothering sort of way but in a medical sort of way. When my friends or neighbors would get injuries or become ill, I would patch them up and take care of them. After high school I became a paramedic. I worked my way up to Critical Care Flight Paramedic working on an Air Ambulance Helicopter.

In February of 2001, I was covering for a coworker who was out on maternity leave when we got called for a heart attack patient on an oilrig. While we were flying out to the oil rig to pick up our patient, I was communicating with the medics on the oil rig, finding out the status of the patient and what he needed. I was getting my medications ready and my cardiac monitor/defibrillator. While I was doing this, I noticed that my fellow crewmembers were tightening their seat belts. I looked up at the Pilot, he looked back at me. I could see the fear in his eyes. I saw the master warning light flashing on the dashboard of the helicopter. I didn't even have time to put my helmet on before we crashed.

I didn't hear any sound when we crashed. I remember the crash. We landed in the forest, in the tops of the trees. I could smell the jet fuel leaking. Our pilot was telling us to get out but we couldn't. When we crashed into the trees, a somewhat small branch (about four inches in diameter) penetrated the helicopter door and impaled me. The branch went right into by lower left abdomen, shattered my pelvic bones and exited through my left hip area narrowly missing my kidney. I was now hooked to this wrecked helicopter that was leaking fuel and smoking. The pilot and other Flight medic worked together to break the branch so we could get out of the helicopter. I only felt the first three kicks at the branch. The pilot helped me out of the aircraft and into the trees. The next thing I remember is the rescue helicopter.

I woke up six weeks later in the hospital. I was being wheeled down a hallway. I remember looking up at the ceiling tiles and saying how filthy the tiles were. "They told us you wouldn't make it but you did it". I had been in a coma for six weeks, had three surgeries and received over 400 stitches and over 200 staples. I had a fractured pelvis, broken ribs, broken ankles, my nose was almost ripped from my face, broken jaw, teeth and now lot and lots of scars. I felt like Frankenstein's Bride.

After my recovery and being home for a while, I tried going back to work in the helicopter. Then every time we had the slightest bit of turbulence I was scared and in a panic. It scared my patients and I realized I wasn't serving my patients well. I was feeling very low. I had scars all over, I couldn't do my job effectively and now I really was not pretty. I felt hopeless.

My sister was constantly telling me that I was pretty and beautiful. I didn't believe her. I have never thought of myself as pretty, beautiful or even sexy. She took me to a Hooters Restaurant this one day and was telling me how pretty I was. I was tired of hearing it because I just didn't believe it. So, to shut her up, I requested the manager of the restaurant. When he arrived at our table, I asked him "am I pretty enough to be a Hooters Girl?" He looked me up and down then said "you're hired". I was so set on hearing him say "no" that I didn't even hear his answer at first.

I was just too busy gloating to my sister to realize I had just been hired to work at Hooters.

Since then so many wonderful things have been happening for me. While I was working at Hooters, I received an offer to be a cover girl for a well-known cosmetic company. I became a Playboy Bunny and worked at the Palms Casino in Las Vegas Nevada. I have worked several commercials a television series and a small part in Hangover Part III.

It has been an incredible, tough and stressful journey. When I was in the hospital they were feeding me with a tube, since I was lying down for months and months I gained lots of weight. So I had lots of scars, low self-esteem, I lost my career and massive weight gain. I asked myself; what do I have left? I cried all the time, felt sorry for myself, and figured what's the point. Then one morning while I was throwing myself a pity party it was like a light bulb was turned on. I realized that I had been given a gift. A gift to live my life again. But this time to do it better. Best of all it was up to me…just me.

I started to exercise by simply riding my bike around the block. Nothing major, not the tour de France, just a simple bike ride. And you know what, I HAD FUN. Then I started to watch what I ate. No science stuff, no fad diets, no "magic" pills. I just watched my calories. I set a limit of calories and stuck to it. Imagine my excitement when I started to lose weight. I started using my moisturizers on my skin, taking care of my hair, and just being good to myself. I found out that life in itself is a gift. None of us know when it will end and it is up to us to make life a wonderful ride. I did this and you can too.

To this very day, I still watch what I eat. I now ride my bike 20 miles per day. I do 100 sit-ups every morning 6 days a week. I don't let life's little problems get me down as there are some things that we just can't change. I have never had a bad day that did not turn out pretty good in the long run. Even my scars have started to fade.

I went from being a crash survivor, to Frankenstein's bride, to a credited Actress, Pin up Model and Playboy bunny. I survived when everyone said I wouldn't, if I can get through this, then you could get through anything too. ENJOY THE GIFT OF LIFE.

Abigail Rich

I started my career being as a Flight Paramedic and through a series of twists an turns as only life can provide, I became an actress and model.

Never Say "I Wish"... Make it Happen
by Katie Rowlett

I have been an athlete my entire life. From grade school all the way up until the day I walked across that stage and received my college degree I have been digging to the depths of pushing beyond what I thought I was capable of, staying focused on a goal, and being disciplined. All in all my years in athletics and competing has been one of the most rewarding aspects of my life. I have learned very valuable life lessons through it all. I have learned that there is no such thing as chance.

To go from an "I wish" to making it happen you must not think about the things you can't do but instead, you need to focus and think about the things you CAN. To remember that NO matter what the level of your ability, you have more potential than you could ever develop in a lifetime. Holding on to the truth that you have powers you never dreamed of and that you can do things you never thought you could do will pave the way to achieving the goals you set for yourself. There are no limitations to what you can do except the limitations of your own mind.

I truly believe all I have achieved in my life is because I lived my life with the firm belief that I CAN have or do anything I want, if I want it bad enough. If I visualize, plan, commit and then do, it WILL happen, NO EXCUSES! This way of believing is one that you can adopt and live by too!

Adopting this belief is just the beginning. Living it out day by day with NO FINISH LINE in sight is where the true success happens. As I mentioned before, you have more potential than you could ever develop in a lifetime, so use your entire lifetime to try and develop all that you can and the only way to do that is to keep going believing that there is no finish line. Every day is a day to improve, to listen and to work hard. There will be no end in sight. Every day is a gift, and what we do with it is our gratitude and gift given in return.

I have been blessed beyond my desires when it comes to the life I have lead up until this point and I am not just talking about my athletic and fitness career. Because of the attitudes and beliefs I am sharing with you, becoming and staying committed and determined from start to finish on the task at hand, I have achieved success in all genres of my life.

No, I am not arrogant enough to say that I have not been through trials and tribulations that have completely wiped me out, but with those hard times, I have learned more about life and myself than I ever would have in all my winning moments. Life is a test and if you can stay focused, visualize and never cease to strive to reach the goals you set out to achieve, SUCCESS will be YOURS!

Whatever your journey maybe or consist of, sooner or later if you are serious enough, you will go through a special, very personal experience that will be only unique to you. It may be a certain failure, a goal or you just are ready to start living the life you were intended to live. Whatever it may be, that is when you will be overcome by a flash of determination, a sense of purpose and drive. It's a new kind of mystical experience that propels you into an elevated state of consciousness.

The experience is unique to each of us, but when it happens you break through a barrier that separates you from the casual person. Forever. And from that point on, there is no finish line. You train for life. You begin to be addicted to what working out and training gives you. When you get here then you can then stop saying "I wish" and MAKE IT HAPPEN!

This life is about you and your story. Only you are capable of writing a story that you can be proud of. Get out of your own way and step up to that starting line and START living out the successful life we all were meant to have. Success will be unique to all of us, but either way or whatever it looks like to you, get going and know that you are on a journey with no finish line.

Beating the competition is relatively easy. But beating yourself is a never ending commitment. There is no finish line, so enjoy the journey!

Katie Rowlett

I am in LOVE with LIFE and am on this journey with the hopes to inspire and change as many lives as God sees fit along the way. I want to share the passion, drive and desire that I have discovered through Fitness!

Having Faith in Your Surroundings
by Jill Rudison

You are today exactly where you are supposed to be...

In competing, I have discovered that I am constantly learning more about myself, who I am and what makes me tick with the completion of every contest. This year was the most bittersweet of my competition career and I wanted to share my story of how the best day of my life was also one of my darkest. Looking back now, I truly believe that everything that transpired on that day was a direct result of fate, and it ultimately taught me that I am far stronger than I will ever even fully realize.

I FINALLY won my Pro Card in Physique Bodybuilding at the IFBB North Americans in Pittsburgh, PA. Not only did I win my card and my class, but I also went on to win the Open Physique Overall title and walk away the big winner of the division. Happily, my folks were there to witness it, there in my father's hometown of Pittsburgh, which obviously meant A LOT to me to have them see it all go down first-hand in my dad's old stomping grounds. It was the most memorable of shows and also the most forgettable – only because it seemed to fly by SO fast and everything felt dream-like and "pinch me" kind of surreal. The 24 hours that led up to the show were INSANE to put it mildly, and I learned more about myself that day/night than I had known for years. Needless to say, it was an extremely bittersweet 24 hours.

Before athlete check-in that afternoon as I was waiting in the lobby of the hotel to be spray tanned, I got a message from a friend that rattled me to the core and broke my heart in two. My dear friend and pseudo big-brother Jed had chosen to take his young life that very morning. As I read the message I sat stunned – in utter disbelief in what I was reading and heartbroken that I hadn't spoken to him before he chose to leave this Earth. Every emotion I was feeling that day – sadness, nervousness, anger, frustration, fear and anxiety swelled up in the back of my throat and ultimately exploded out of my mouth as gallons of tears began to stream from my eyes. I got up, blurted out to my coach and friend Chris Cormier that Jed had died and ran for the doors. I pushed open the lobby doors and exploded onto the sidewalk outside, hysterically crying and still trying to process that my friend was gone. I had just spoken to him. We had plans to hang out when I got home. He promised me that I was going to win this show, get my Pro card and come home a winner. I was crestfallen and numb. I felt like the world had just been yanked out from underneath my feet. I had been on such a high that to suddenly hear this news…it absolutely devastated me. I felt broken. I didn't want to do anything except cry and die myself. I felt helpless.

If it hadn't of been for Chris and Marilyn from Liquid Sun Rayz, I would have collapsed into a puddle of Jill on the floor. They truly were amazing to me at that awful moment and for that I am FOREVER grateful. As I stood in the tanning booth, buck nekkid, water-depleted and being sprayed a beautiful bronze hue, I quietly laughed through my tears only because I knew that Jed was looking down at me at that very moment, probably both mortified and amused at my nekkidness and of the scene in general. (If you compete, you KNOW how WEIRD a tanning area looks for a competition. It's freaking BIZARRE.) Strangely, that provided me with some comfort and my innate ability to somehow find humor in an otherwise sick and twisted situation. But that was Jed, and this is me, and we always had the same dark sense of humor, so I found peace in that. And standing there being sprayed orange, I decided that I had NO choice but to win the show not only for me, but to keep my promise to my friend. I had a lengthy mental conversation with Jed during that hour, and knew that my failure, for once, was absolutely NOT an option this time around.

After leaving the hotel, I drove across the bridge and checked in at the host hotel. Easy enough, right? I checked in, said hello to a friend, and was in and out within minutes. I then left the hotel with the intention of driving straight back to my hotel by the University and laying in bed with my legs elevated the rest of the night. Instead I offered to pick up Chris at another hotel he was at to see a client, and somehow ended up SO lost that I found myself literally stranded in the middle of "Nowheresville" for 2 hours. Now, considering the news I had just gotten, my multiple days of water and carb depletion, being 3 hours late for a meal and stressed, I was not in what you would call a 'happy place'. After a million U-turns, gas station stops, tears, and epic temper tantrum phone calls to Chris to somehow come save me, he managed to do just that. Annnnnd then he proceeded to get us lost for another hour and a half. LOL

When we FINALLY made it back to the hotel, I scarfed down some food, quickly settled in for the night and got my bag ready for the morning. I didn't fall asleep easily that night…my brain was too overloaded to fully relax. Instead I lay in bed and replayed my last visit with Jed just a few weeks earlier at my house. He had been in such good spirits and seemed genuinely happy. So much so, that I offered to give him a key to my place to come over and bask on the sundeck anytime he wanted. He loved my little backyard and I now find great comfort sitting out there and thinking about my friend. I kick myself in the ass EVERY day that I didn't get to chat with him before he chose to leave us, or that I didn't do more or "sense" more was going on with him prior to his last few days. It will be a regret that I will carry the rest of my life. I still struggle with his absence…reaching for the phone to text him when I see something funny in the world of MMA, or calling him to come over and hang out or even just thinking "oh, I should invite Jed"…only to slowly realize that I can't do that anymore. His absence has left a gaping hole in my heart that I doubt will ever be filled again. Probably not. He was truly one of a kind and one of the most gentle and genuinely "feeling" people I have ever met.

The next day I was eerily calm. I knew I had a mission to complete and I was laser-precision focused. If I could get through the last 24 hours of crazy my life, I was ready to tackle the world. Blindfolded. Handcuffed even.

After I got my hair & makeup done and was suited up and ready to go, we left for the Sheraton. I felt eerily confident in my abilities and was calm in knowing that I had truly given it my all and felt 200% ready to take the stage. I also knew that I had a newly appointed guardian angel looking over me – one who was more badass than most others – and I knew that I would have the heavens shining down on me that day.

Now, I'm not religious by ANY means, but I will admit that I am spiritual. And I wholeheartedly knew that with Jed's spirit by my side, I could achieve anything I set out to that day. Before I knew it, I was taking out my curlers and running onstage with Chris still trying to glaze my legs and back up, with almost 8 months of full prep leading up to that moment. I took a few deep breaths, smiled like a used-car salesman and walked out on stage. The judges had us do our mandatory poses and began to move competitors around like chess pieces. I didn't even realize that I hadn't been moved at all myself, just everyone moving in circles around me, and only after I came off stage did I realize that I had been holding down the coveted middle spot on stage. Once that was pointed out to me, I couldn't contain my happiness and grinned ear to ear for the rest of the day. We schlepped back to our hotel where I took a much-deserved and extremely restful nap before waking up to re-curl my hair and again head out to the Sheraton Hotel.

That's when everything became a super fast FLASH of blurred

memories. I remember taking out my curlers, lining up, doing my routine, and being pulled into the top 5 line up. I went out on stage beaming with pride and personal satisfaction and remember squeezing my poses SO hard that all I could hear was myself mentally yelling "Squeeze! Squeeze! Squeeze!" and Jed's voice yelling "War Team Rudison!!" – his personal war cry he had created for my shows. They began counting down the winner from 5th place, and after 2nd place was called I realized that I had FINALLY done it. I had finally won my class and finally won that damn IFBB Pro Card that I had only dreamed about for soooo long. After I won my class I walked off stage (felt more like floating, actually) and flew into the arms of Chris who greeted me with open arms, tears and excited cries. We spun around and around, jumping and crying and making a complete scene and before I knew it I was again being sent out on stage to compete for the Open Overall title. Again, I stood on stage like frozen Han Solo, until someone nudged me to walk forward and receive the coveted Overall trophy. I didn't even know how to properly receive the trophy or do a victory pose, because I had never until that very moment been "victorious". I was in absolute bliss. I have never in my life been 1st Place at a NPC show, much less an Overall Winner and now a bonafide Pro athlete. I was stunned and shocked and truly needed someone to pinch me until I bled because I still couldn't believe it.

And I STILL cannot believe it.

Immediately afterwards I did numerous backstage interviews and got congratulated by peers, fans, fellow competitors and chairpersons. I was on such a HIGH, I never wanted to come down. To have what I have known as being the WORST feeling in the world suddenly turn the tide into what I can only describe as the BEST feeling in the world is such a mind fuck. People always talk about the highs and lows of life and how fragile and delicate it is, and I can honestly say that I absolutely did not know this feeling until that very day. I am one of "those" people who believe that things happen for a reason - both good and bad - and that we are where we are supposed to be, learning and experiencing the things we are supposed to, when we are supposed to. I believe that people come into your life for very specific reasons and that even things that seem to be simple acts of randomness and chance, are indeed pre-disposed to happen to us, no matter how small or insignificant they may seem at the time. I know that my friendship with Jed was meant to be, just as much as I struggle to accept that he chose to leave when he did. I also believe that it was finally MY time to be victorious and my fate awarded me so.

After the show, I stayed behind a few days to check out the Andy Warhol Museum and visit with family I hadn't seen in over 20 years. We had a great reunion with family in the lower bottoms of McKees Rocks, eating a ton of food, telling a ton of stories and somehow NOT taking any photos. (Ugh. The conversation was just too good, I suppose.) My cousin Shawn pulled me to the side and told me the sweetest story about how I hadn't changed a BIT since I was a little kid. He laughed at how I had blossomed into a (muscular) woman, yet still somehow managed to retain the SAME laser-point precision and focus he said I have possessed since childhood. He swears I still have the same crinkle in my forehead and eerie stare I used to muster up at times when I was determined to set out and achieve a goal or prove someone wrong. 27 years may have passed, but he maintains that the little girl with the laser-precision stare still lives within me. I absolutely loved hearing that. And I love that I still am the SAME person I have been all of my life. I'm just more evolved and wiser.

The next day I returned to LA to everything being completely different, yet still exactly the same. I'm constantly being asked how it feels to be a Pro now and people seem truly alarmed when I say that it feels exactly the same as it did when I was an amateur. (Well, it does!)

Miriam Khalladi

The only blaring difference now is that I have to work twice as hard, if not three times as hard, since I am now standing shoulder to shoulder with the best of the best. So, I guess to be 100% honest in answering the question, as much as everything shall change, everything shall remain exactly the same; Laser-point precision stares, friendships, victory poses, the sun shining on my back deck…the only difference is how you feel about it.

And these days I feel pretty grateful about life…

For you, Jed Abrams. Thank you for allowing me to know true friendship for the brief time you graced me with yours. See you on the flipside.

RIP 8/30/12

Jill Rudison
I'm a full-time IFBB Physique Pro, part-time producer & All-The-Time Bad Ass.

Get Out of Your Own Way
by Cassandra Sawyer

Can I just be honest, and put it out there? Real Talk, Real Women… well here you go!

I was struggling. Struggling badly! When approached to be a contributor to this book, I instantly accepted and was humbled by the opportunity. I thought about what a great platform I was being given to share all the motivational energy, perspective and ability I had swirling around inside. But, as I sat down to put pen to paper, I didn't freeze, I regressed! I wish it was simple writers' block that plagued me, but something even worse took over….fear. All of a sudden, doubt flooded my mind and I wasn't sure I had anything to share anymore. I wasn't sure if anyone would care. I wasn't sure if I would be as good as the other women contributing to the book.

I was able to punch out a few lines every day and after several weeks was getting close to achieving the minimum word count requested. But I just wasn't moved by anything I wrote. There was no conviction. More or less, it represented me and my perspective, but it just felt like words on paper. At T-minus 48 hours to the deadline I was seriously contemplating responding that while I appreciate the offer, I just don't think I'm what this book needs. It was going to kill me to quit, but I'd rather not be in the book, than be substandard in the book. At T-minus 24 hours, I did my weekly track workout and almost hyperventilated because I was crying while running, wondering what am I going to do. How many opportunities would I get in life to be a part of such an amazing group of women? I wanted this so bad, but I just couldn't come up with anything worthwhile. After an hour and fifteen minutes of running, sprints, lunges and stair climbs I lay spent in the middle of a football field mentally drafting my email response. Then I realized that what I was prepared to say declining this offer, is exactly what I should say in my chapter. The book is called Real Talk, Real Women…well this is pretty real, as far as I'm concerned and is at the heart of my desire to even have a platform.

As I've grown in fitness and in life, I've learned more about myself in those "weak" moments that in any other time. As I've recognized that I CAN push past a difficult moment, learn, grow and thrive as a result, I have come to enjoy pushing myself to my limits. I have learned that feeling weak, doesn't make you weak. In fact, the opposite is quite often the outcome. You become stronger (physically and mentally), wiser and now have the added value of an experience that no one can take away from you. I feel like I stumbled upon the Holy Grail with this lesson! A lesson that as a wife and mother have seen others and have personally myself, circumvented because I thought I had to for my family. This is obviously not true and is at the foundation of the reason why I put myself out there….the good, the bad, the sweaty ugly and the vulnerably nervous, to hopefully demonstrate the gift you are giving by challenging yourself to take risks and live the life of your dreams. Yes, people are counting on you. But don't forget that you are one of them.

I have felt that it would be too hard on me and my family to do a variety of things… go back to school to get my MBA, find time to work out to compete, spend money on healthy organic food to cook each night, to earn my PHR and CPT certifications, the list goes on and on. But each of these accomplishments has not only provided me a sense of pride and accomplishment, but they are real life examples of the challenges I want my children to take on. And what a blessing is the benefit of seeing and knowing that they can achieve anything they want to achieve. To my children, I want to say, do as I say AND as I do. Doubt will come and that is ok. Feel the fear and do it anyway. And as a matter of fact, the instant you recognize fear is trying to hold you back, accept that as life's challenge to you. A test to earn the glory that lives on the other side of fear.

As I lay there on the grass, I gave thought to how I would feel in 10, 20, 30 or 50 years from now, if I didn't write this chapter. Immediately a sense of grief hit me. My heart hurt and it felt like I was mourning the loss of something. This is often the barometer I use to make big and small decisions in my life. The fact is that those days will come. God willing, I will reach 10, 20, 30 and 50 years from now and look back on my life to that point. What am I going to feel and think? Am I going to get that sense of mourning and loss over not even trying to achieve my goals? Or is my heart going warm at the memories of what appeared insurmountable at the time, now just a sense of pride? Will a smile break across my face recalling the trivial "obstacles" and even legitimate challenges presented that I chose to overcome? Well, I know that if I experience grief now over the thought, I will definitely experience grief over the reality. How unnecessary. Regret has to be one of the most painful feelings to live with, because it means you had a choice and the power over the outcome. I find it hard to truly regret the knowledge that comes with life lessons. However, I do regret what I haven't been brave enough to try.

Eventually, I got up and brushed myself off…physically and mentally. I walked back to my car with a sense of purpose, reminded that no matter how exhausted I was, I was the only person who could drive me to where I wanted to be. I refused to get a copy of this book and not be in it. I would, of course, applaud and congratulate the other ladies, but I am not a great spectator.

I don't have what it takes to sit back and watch. I need to be active participants in life, making things happen for myself. This is part of the reason I don't enjoy watching sports, reality competition or awards shows on TV. For some this is an enjoyable escape from reality. For me it a reminder that there are people out there right now actively pursuing their dreams, and I should be one of them. They are putting in the work while I watch. When someone wins, I am happy for them because it is a demonstration that hard work does pay off, but it is not my win. I didn't earn it. I long for the celebration that accompanies the satisfaction of achievement from hard work that I put in. The pleasure that comes from accomplishing a goal is unparalleled. Maybe even addictive. To get your fix, you must set a new goal. I'm ok with that!

Well, as I wrap up my contribution to this book, I am at T minus 12 hours before the deadline and happy. I didn't use a single sentence from my original rough draft or even stay on the topic I had planned to write about.

With the sense of purpose and desire I felt to share this experience of getting over fear and doubt, the words flew onto the page in just over an hour. Which included stopping to make a peanut butter and jelly sandwich for my daughter and using the restroom twice, as I'm chasing down my daily gallon of water.

It feels miraculous and is yet another example for me of the incredible things that can be done by simply getting out of your own way.

Cassandra Sawyer
I'm taking fitness mainstream by sharing my passion and uncovering yours!

Success Starts with Happiness
by Andrea Smith

In the summer of 2007, my life changed drastically … I graduated from high school, moved 3,000 miles away to college, and developed an eating disorder that caused a mysterious and drastic weight gain. I was baffled as to why I was gaining all this weight; I thought I was eating well. After consulting with a doctor, I discovered that I had developed sleep-eating disorder, which caused me to sleep walk, and "sleep eat". I would eat foods high in fats, sugars, and bad carbohydrates. The disorder stemmed from feelings that I was suppressing from a very emotionally abusive relationship. I have always had a very small build at 5'5" and 120 lbs., so when I gained 30 plus pounds in a few short months I started to freak out. After finding out the root of all the evil, I tried to take back both my life and my body. Looking for a quick fix, I turned to yo-yo and fad dieting. However, any weight I did lose was gained back, PLUS SOME! This caused even more frustration with my weight, and I became stuck in what seemed like an endless cycle of dieting and gaining what weight I had lost, with an additional ten pounds each time.

In 2009 I weighed in at my highest weight of 176 pounds. I was sick of feeling tired and sluggish, and knew that I needed change. My confidence, happiness, and self-esteem were gone, and with a new man in my life (whom I now call my husband) I wanted to feel attractive and sexy for myself.

I had to change my mind frame because everything I had done in the past had ended in failure. I needed a goal to work towards. I decided on something I was familiar with: A PAGEANT. Pageants were something I had done for 5 years, starting in the seventh grade. I spent months running like a madwoman, eating a low calorie diet and sometimes not eating but once a day. I never thought about the damage I was doing to my body. When I competed in the pageant, I won "Pennsylvania's Prettiest Smile" but not the crown. Although I was proud of myself for giving it my all, I was not happy and knew that participating in pageants was not the answer to my problem. I wanted to lose the weight I gained from my eating disorder. I wanted to be healthy. I wanted my confidence back. I wanted to be proud of myself. Knowing this, I began searching for the answer that would grant me the happiness I knew I deserved.

A year later I stumbled across stories in fitness magazines about women following the clean eating lifestyle with wonderful success. I especially fell in love with Oxygen magazine and came across the success story of fitness inspiration Kelsey Byers. Her determination and passion inspired me. Seeking advice, I sent her an email. In almost no time at all she emailed me back and the moment I received that email I became instantly emotional, crying at my computer because I felt the answers I had been searching for a very long time were now answered. After sending a few more emails back and forth, Kelsey encouraged me to create a fan page to help share my passion and love for fitness and clean eating while helping to inspire others with my story. She directed me towards all of Tosca Reno's books, and I started reading them from cover to cover. I did more research on clean eating, bought tons of fitness magazines, hired a trainer at the gym to show me what and how to lift weights properly. I even purged my apartment kitchen of all "unclean foods." Boy oh boy was my husband in shock. At this point, thanks to Kelsey's advice and friendship, it's safe to say I was finally ready to hop on board the clean eating and weight lifting train!

On September 4, 2011, the day after my wedding, I truly began my journey to a new and improved healthier self. First I wrote a list of all the groceries I needed to buy. Then I reorganized my daily life in such a way that allowed me to be more focused on meal prepping and my workouts. The first two months were the most challenging, but not because of the diet. I was very satisfied by the flavor and the amount of food I was eating. The challenging part was saying "no" to friends asking to go to lunch at Applebee's or Olive Garden, and turning down fruity cocktails, beers, and wine. I will also confess that giving up certain condiments, such as mayo and ranch dressing was difficult, but all I had to do was remember why I had started, and suddenly it became much easier to say "no." After three months of being completely immersed in this new way of living and finding new friends that shared the same interest, I realized how important all of this was to me.

This was my lifestyle. I had begun my fitness journey. Even though I was familiar with working out and exercising, it was necessary that I learned the proper techniques and the science behind building lean muscle and burning fat. Briefly hiring a personal trainer and doing my own research allowed me to find a stronger me. Since I was still just a beginner, I did what my body could take. Cardio, tracking my heart rate, using lighter weights with high repetitions were vital to achieving my new goals. Based off of my growing strength and the changes in my body, I altered my workouts and weight training sessions.

It took about three months for me to start seeing results and get my metabolism back to where it should have been. During this time it is safe to say my husband became annoyed hearing any self-doubt I had, which I often expressed by saying things like "Why am I doing this? I'm NOT seeing results! I haven't lost anything!" He remained supportive through it all and never let me give up. It was difficult to push through those first few months, and it took all I had to NOT set foot on the scale.

About a month later, when I was four months into eating clean and lifting weights, other people started seeing change in not only my body, but in my confidence. That's when they started asking me about what I had been doing. It was then that I realized that my new lifestyle was impacting those around me. People were noticing that my hard work was paying off! I loved hearing comments from friends and family like "You look amazing! Tell me about your new lifestyle." Losing 15 pounds in only 3 months was such an accomplishment, and I was so proud of myself. This was when my mind starting wandering, dreaming, and setting new goals. I'm the type of person who needs goals to focus on, so I began writing down short and long term goals to hang on my vision boards, bathroom mirror, and in my daily fitness journal so I could be reminded of them every day. This is when I took Kelsey Byers' advice to start a fan page on Facebook. My fan page became a way for me to inspire, motivate, and help others find the information I once was searching for. I believe if I can help inspire or motivate one person then everything is worth it.

After two years of hard work, dedication to the clean eating lifestyle, and undergoing the removal of my gallbladder, I've never felt so proud and empowered by who I am now! Since my lifestyle and mindset have changed I can honestly say I've never been so happy with who I am and where I am going. There was never a magical number on the scale or clothing size I wanted to achieve. I just wanted to feel healthy and fit; to accomplish the better vision I had of myself.

I am more gratified not with what I've lost, but what I had gained. I had become emotionally sound, spiritually centered, and mentally healthier. Fitness and clean eating had not only transformed my body, but also completely changed my life.

If I could share one secret that helped me to be successful in reaching my goals and continuing to strive for more it would be that what I did is NOT a diet. It is, however, a LIFESTYLE, which is something you must be ready to take on without looking back to the "old" you for comfort.

This lifestyle is something that you must be ready for because it's challenging, demanding, and requires an open mind. You must be open to a whole new beginning and a whole new you! It wasn't until I DECIDED to make small differences, each and every day, adding them all together, that I achieved my goal and lost 50lbs.

Andrea Smith
I'm an esthetician. Marine Wife. Fitness Inspiration. Fitness Model. Health Coach. Living Proof Gear Ambassador. 50lbs weight loss success story with a passion to help others achieve their goals.

Life is Full of Detours
by Nikki Stelzer

Setbacks Don't Showcase Your Weaknesses, They Develop Your Strengths.

I was 27 and engaged to the man of my dreams. I was loving life and feeling as if each day was better than the next. How could life possibly get any better? We both had great jobs and met at the perfect time in our lives. It seemed like all the stars had aligned and my life was in complete balance. So naturally, what did I have to do? Shake things up of course! Instead of living in the moment I couldn't help but think of the next thing, the next thing, the next thing, and how'd I plan for it.

Babies! I swear getting married makes your biological clock tick really loud for everyone to hear. I couldn't have a single conversation about my husband and I without them asking when I was having a baby. Which got me thinking….my husband is 7 years older than me and my dad was 75 at the time, maybe they are right? What am I waiting for!? So I began questioning everything. How am I going to balance my career and family? Am I going to want to be a stay at home mom? Wait no, I'll go crazy being a stay at home mom. Right? Than who will watch my kids? Is daycare really safe? If I stay home for a few years will my career pass me by? Hold on, do I even like my job?

I was at a point in my career where it was difficult to get to the next level at my relatively young age and I was getting inpatient (go figure). I was working hard, putting in the hours but my turn hadn't come yet. How could I be a good mom and work at this pace to get to the next level? Besides, is there really such a thing as having it all? I was scared that it wasn't all possible; something had to give, right? So I left the only industry I knew and put the last 8 years of my career behind me.

I decided that I wanted a more "flexible job" and the potential to run my own business one day. So I took an opportunity in PR and Marketing. All of a sudden I was working 12+ hour days, including weekends and holidays! It was so crazy that I would forget to eat and drink during work and was too busy to sleep, exercise, or spend time with my husband when I got home. What had I done!

I knew this new job wasn't for me but I didn't want to admit that I may have made a mistake. I was convinced that I couldn't go back to my prior career and I was too proud and embarrassed to ask for my old job back, so I took a job at a small no name firm to get back into the finance industry. What a mistake that was! If it took me 6 weeks to realize the last marketing job wasn't for me, it seemed like only 6 minutes passed before I wanted to bail on this one too. Improvement I suppose?

How did I get myself here? I felt hopeless and defeated and wanted to avoid all contact with my friends and former colleagues because inevitably they'd ask how work was going. I couldn't bear to tell them I had 3 jobs in the last 4 months! I was supposed to be the stable, sensible one in the group.

Finally I got the courage to talk about my situation with a close friend and confidant. I will never forget our conversation. She said, "Nikki, why are you planning for a baby that's not even here yet? When that time comes, do what is best for you and your husband; at that moment! Don't get caught up in planning for the what-ifs and the maybes, because when we plan God laughs. Just focus on the here and now." She went on to try and convince me to ask for my old job back. I appreciated the wise words and decided to start applying to companies in my prior line of work, but not my old firm.

Yea, still too stubborn. I couldn't possible take ALL of her advice at once. I still wanted to hold on to my pride and figure things out for myself.

Once I gained my confidence back I was lining up interviews but nothing seemed like the right fit for me. One night, after another long talk with my friend I decide to contact my old boss. Turns out they just filled my old position and the person was moving down that week to take my old job! I was too late. Why didn't I just swallow my pride and call them sooner when I realized things weren't working out as planned? Well they say that fate will find a way.... I still owe Fate a bundle for introducing me to my husband, but it seems she came through again. I got a phone call from a former colleague saying they were hiring for my old position at the office near my house!

In the end I got my old job back and my life has returned to "normal". The difference now is that I count all my blessing and remember these 10 valuable life lessons that this setback taught me:

1. When life is sailing along smoothly, don't make waves! Appreciate the calm while it lasts.
2. Be careful what you wish for! Things don't always turn out the way you planned.
3. Live life on your own terms, on your own timetable. Don't give into the pressures of society.
4. Don't be too stubborn to admit your mistakes or too proud to learn from them.
5. Don't let a setback showcase your weaknesses; let it develop your strengths.
6. Have at least one friend that is older and much wiser; listen when they speak!
7. Fate doesn't ask what you want; it knows what's best even if when you don't.
8. Sometimes we need to take a step back to see what's right in front of us.

9. Planning creates great roadmaps; just know that life is full of detours. Enjoy the journey.
10. 1A setback is only as long as the time it takes to get back on your feet. So pick yourself up and try again!

Nikki Stelzer

I'm a lifelong cheerleader, treadmill racer, eternal optimist, passionate volunteer, thrill seeker and lover of all things pink!

The Road to Recovery
by Amy von Rummelhoff

I never thought I'd get a shot at the pro card. Stepping on stage last July at the NPC USA's in Las Vegas was both nerve-racking and exhilarating. I can still remember my growing anticipation as I stood under the bright lights, waiting for my number to be called. The carpeted stage made one out of three girls trip, and my worries mounted: Would I stumble? Would I turn beet red? Would people laugh?

After 2.5 months of dieting and training, here it was: my moment. I took center stage, eased through my three poses, flashed the judge a smile, and walked off with a sense of relief. I'd ranked in the top 10. Not only was I a trainer, athlete, and fitness model, but I was now a National Level Bikini competitor.

Standing there, I looked like the poster child of health, but I was used to that. As a child, I'd dance for 10 years and taken my passion for figure skating all the way to Nationals. I've always been an athlete. But I've also always had an inner struggle, too.

Recognizing My Difficult Start

From childhood, a weak immune system paired with chronic migraines and asthma kept me on what felt like a million medications. While doctors tried concocting the best medicinal cocktail, my metabolism suffered, causing weight fluctuations and hormonal imbalance. As a kid, I felt frustrated. I wasn't able to run more than ¼ of a lap around the track and remember disapproving looks from my teammates when I was left wheezing on the soccer field.

By high school, I had changed. I took to the rink and traded in the extra pudge for the bumps and bruises that came with competitive figure skating. Asthma flare-ups made it difficult to increase the intensity, but I was determined. I'd become extremely good at ignoring pain - a trait that got me in trouble at age 19.

During midterms week my sophomore year, I managed to ignore a ruptured appendix for four days. It started on a Wednesday morning, when a busy schedule led me to brush off severe flu symptoms and stomach pain as mere stress. I pushed through Thursday, but, when I woke up Friday morning, I was in excruciating pain. Because of all the toxins running through my system, it took nearly ten hours for doctors make a diagnosis.

I woke up to an abscess, an overall drop in health, and a long road to recovery.

Over the next few weeks, I was hooked up to 11 IVs and unable to eat or drink. I trudged through finals on high amounts of painkillers and had someone else carry my backpack because I was too weak. By the time hospital checkout rolled around, I had lost 30 pounds. At 5'9, I weighed in just shy of 110lbs.

Rethinking My "Thin" Obsession

My weight loss was all people could talk about. Guys started hitting on me, and girls spread rumors of eating disorders. I felt conflicted. I knew I was in the worst health of my life, but, having always been frustrated with being the "big girl," it felt good to be skinny - even if it was for the wrong reasons.

When I started putting the weight back on, I freaked out. My "skinny clothes" were tight, and I feared I'd look like I did before. I felt trapped. When I was stress, sad, or depressed, I would restrict or binge and purge. The only way I knew to numb the pain was to empty my body - throwing up anything I thought was bad or not eating at all.

I never had a distinct moment of enlightenment, but I slowly realized that if I didn't make a change, I'd never know what it felt like to be healthy. I was tired of over exercising and of my strict "diet." I'd had enough.

Embracing My Budding Recovery

I made baby steps towards recovery, but it was a constant battle. I would start counting the days I was "good," but then I'd get a migraine or stress would kick in, and I'd relapse. In the beginning, I focused on eating protein with every meal and consuming more greens. I worked out 4-5 days a week but didn't understand the importance of weight training and did more cardio than necessary. I didn't really get on track until my move to LA in 2010.

Moving opened many doors. Within the first four months, I'd landed a production job and booked an infomercial. Soon after, I was training at Jackie Warner's private gym in Beverly Hills. I fueled my passion for fitness by getting certified and training clients.

Being surrounded by people who lived a lifestyle of healthy eating, weight training, and competing, motivated me. After watching all of my fitness friends take the stage, I decided I wanted to prove to myself by training for a competition. I learned how to train and eat right. I found a coach and set a target goal of 8 weeks till I hit the stage.

The diet was strict, but I chocked it up as part of the competition process. I ate five meals of 25 grams of lean protein a day - roughly the size of a small chicken breast. Veggies were fine, but fruits, starchy carbs, dairy, and fats were all off of my diet. I did full body circuits and one hour of steady cardio 5 days a week. My body responded quickly. I learned that I actually liked the structure and that it gave me a healthy sense of control, but I often felt drained.

Confronting My Competitive Downfall

Hard work paid off when I placed 3rd and qualified for the USA's, but that meant no rest, no cheats, and no free time. I was back in the gym Sunday morning training for two hours a day. The thrill of competing on a National stage masked some of the fatigue, and I was able to drag through the next week knowing I was in the home stretch... or so I thought.

I placed 9th, which left me hungry for more.

I had to step up my game. I took no time off from the gym or dieting and pushed to enhance my "lean physique." Then, my body hit a wall. I started feeling puffy and unprepared for my upcoming show. Despite my coach's encouragement, I lacked confidence. When I finished just shy of the top 5, I wished I had listened to my gut and dropped out. I started to gain weight and nothing helped to take it off.

Uncovering My Fitness Hurdle

Eventually, a doctor told me I had metabolic damage. The same "starvation diet" of no carbs or fats that had led to fast results initially had gone on too long, and my metabolism had slowed down to compensate for the lack of nutrients. Instead of burning 2100 calories throughout the day, I dropped to roughly 1000 calories - making weight gain extremely easy and leaving me susceptible to side effects like exhaustion, sensitivity to cold, poor digestion, and bloating.

Reframing My Perspective

I was devastated but decided to push forward. Although I knew the process of trying to rebuild my metabolism would take time and not give the fast results I was hoping for I decided to go for it. Today my body is starting to respond and my body composition is shifting. I am slowly building more muscle while decreasing my body fat %. I am still not satisfied with where I am and I still get frustrated from time to time with all the health battles I fight daily but I just have to tell myself its all part of the journey. The headaches, the constant sickness and the metabolic issues, that's all a part of what makes me me. Nothing has ever come easy for me so why should it start now right? When I finally can look in the mirror and maintain a physique I feel proud of it will be that much more worth it know what I went through to get there.

I recently moved to Boise, ID to manage the female-inspired supplement line FitMiss powered by MusclePharm and met a trainer experienced in working with metabolic issues. We're meticulously working to change up my macros (carbs, fats and protein ratios) to a level my body will respond to. I am training less but at higher intervals, weights and circuits. My cardio is nothing but HIIT cardio and I am slowly increasing my carbs to reverse the carb sensitivity I have developed.

I've set a bigger goal: I want to inspire other women that they too can overcome obstacles and still achieve amazing results the healthy way. Drastic measures don't last, and waking up every morning to chase the beloved pro card can put you off track. It's important to take the occasional step back from your competition bubble and think about why you started your journey in the first place. I do plan to take the stage again next year with a stronger better physique so stay tuned!

Amy von Rummelhoff
I'm a Cali girl, ex competitive figure skater, fitness model and trainer, NPC bikini competitor and entrepreneur.

Hard Work, Passion & Perseverance
by Jen Wenk

A man behind me at the neighborhood Starbucks decides to start some light conversation. Already half-turned with arms folded, he tosses it to me. "Soooo….What kind of work do you do?"

I hesitate but, ok, today I'll give a real answer because why not, I kind of feel like burning some time too. I turn around. He's not into MMA. I checked that at the door. My guy is like 50 or 51, somewhere around there. He wears a grey scissor cut under a faded Nike cap. He's a BBFF, a basketball-baseball-football fan…and sometimes he watches boxing. Definitely.

"I own a public relations agency specializing in combat sports," I say.

His reaction is textbook. For a non-MMA guy. Surprise replaces his smile and I'm hit with a blank stare. He looks me down, then up, and searches for a make-sense reply. Yes this is a woman standing before him, she's petite, kinda feminine looking. Did she really just say combat sports?

We both step forward in the line. "Basically its handling media, special events, publicity and stuff like that for MMA, Muay Thai and kickboxing," I offer.

"Oh like for boxing?"

I shake my head. "No, no. Not like boxing. Like the U-F-C. I spell it out for him. His smile returns.

"Ohhh the UFC. That's that crazy wrestling stuff in the cage, right? That's where the guys fight without rules and are always getting hurt. It's so dangerous. I tried watching it once. It's brutal."

It's my turn to smile. Starbucks buddy has just sent me back to the year 2005. And 2006. And 2007. When my boss Dana White and me are sitting at the desk of a big sports editor. Any editor. Any newspaper. Any one of those years. And he has just said THE EXACT SAME THING to us. To the best of my memory those 05-07 conversations went something like this:

"Well I sure appreciate you coming all the way down here, but we just don't cover the cage fighting stuff. We know it's entertaining and popular. But it's violent. We stick to sports here."

Dana shifts in his chair and leans forward, and his eyes lock in before he starts to engage.

"Yeah, that's one of the most common misperceptions about our sport. People think it's violent," Dana puts emphasis on 'think'. He leans forward, determined to make his mark. "But that's just because people are uneducated about it. That's why we came down here and why wanted to meet with you.

"The truth is that there's never been a serious injury or death ever in the UFC. The most common injury is a cut or a broken finger. And it's been proven in a study that MMA is safer than boxing. Name any sport that can say the same."

Dana doesn't wait for a reply, "You can't. There are more injuries in high school cheerleading."

He's taken the floor and he's full on MMA 101-ing this now intrigued editor who Dana and I know has been quite comfortable covering just the B-B-F and big boxing fights since he took his job 12 years ago. We know, because I did the research, but this was the case across the whole country.

"The thing about the UFC is that everything you're seeing is already an Olympic sport. MMA is Olympic sports mixed together into one sport, that's why it's called Mixed Martial Arts," he says stressing the "Mixed."

"There's Judo, Tae Kwon Do, Boxing, Grappling, Greco-Roman Wrestling…and our fighters," he cuts himself off. "You know these guys are real athletes - most of them train six-seven hours a day and they come from a college sport. 80 percent of our guys have college degrees and if they weren't fighting they would be accountants or lawyers."

He returns to the point, "What they do is learn all of these different sports and mix them into one. That's what makes it so exciting. There are so many different ways you can win and so many different ways you can lose, and no one discipline is better than another. Not only do you have to learn all of them to be a complete fighter, you have to be able to mix them together."

The editor doesn't interrupt. And neither do I, except to point out that UFC now holds a fights every two to three weeks, generating enough news to satisfy a dedicated beat writer or regular MMA column. And that other major daily newspapers that gave us a shot with trial coverage, reported back that UFC stories ranked among their highest trafficked stories online, if not the highest.

"Yeah our numbers are crazy. Our website does four million uniques a month. Our reality show The Ultimate Fighter is the highest rated show on television with Males 18-42. We are the number one live event on Pay-Per-View and we sell out venues wherever we go. UFC is the fastest growing sport in history, and we're going to become the biggest sport in the world."

Dana's last remark is met by silence. I smile because I know what's coming next for the traditional sports editor who just doesn't cover ultimate fighting.

"I know what you're thinking. But think about this. Fighting is in our DNA. It was the first real sport. If you're walking down the street, and there's basketball on one corner, football on the other, soccer at the third, and then a fight breaks out on the fourth. Where does the crowd go?"

The three of us nod in agreement. "They go to watch the fight."

"That would be true," says the editor.

"It doesn't have to be explained to you. No matter what country you are from or what language you speak, everyone understands fighting. Football is the biggest sport in the United States, no denying that, but the NFL will never be big in Europe. Just like cricket will never be big here. But fighting, fighting transcends all languages and cultural barriers. And as human beings, we get it - and most of us - like it."

Dana's given our subject a lot to think about. After another 15 minutes or so of sports talk and a state of the UFC address, that includes statistics about the exponential growth of fans, Pay-Per-View buys and interest in general, we leave the State to return to Las Vegas and our 24/7 focus on the next fight.

In exactly three days the sports editor will assign one his writers to do a trial preview story. And the next day he'll call me back to say this ultimate fighting thing is pretty popular with readers. He'll ask if I will continue working with his writer on future events. Another wall is knocked down, and we have gained another supporter with influence and power in the media.

I zoom back to 2013 and have just given my coffee line partner this same drill.

To his credit, he returns a thoughtful smile. He doesn't disagree with me. He asks, "Yeah, you know, I should check out a fight sometime. When is the next event?"

I give him information on the next UFC event in Vegas. He grabs his Americana to go and heads out the door. Maybe he was just being nice, but maybe he wasn't. Maybe he will keep an open mind the next time he's sees MMA and give it a chance. Either way, he had more of an education than he did yesterday, and that's why I never ever give up – I never stop continuing the work I started in 2005 with a team of eight and a visionary who to this day is committed to building the biggest sport in the world.

Never Give Up.

Jen Wenk

I'm the founder of StarPR Las Vegas – a PR agency specializing in combat sports, and the former long-time head of PR for the Ultimate Fighting Championship.

Finding Your Passion is Everyone's Quest in Life
by Shannan Yorton Penna

Many people drift through life with no real direction. They go where circumstances take them like a ship without a rudder. And going wherever you are led can be a definite course for disaster as we all have deep internal drives that must be met. If we ignore our deepest passions and instead choose another path, either through inaction or, by taking the path of least resistance we are normally left unfulfilled and feeling like we missed out on a greater purpose.

While deep down most of us know this to be true, others feel that they don't even have something that speaks to them strongly enough that they could call it a passion. What then? Many people ask how do I find my passion? How do I know what that thing is that is going to make me feel completely self-actualized? My mission? My Quest?

Some answers would be, to make time for discovering and finding that passion. Prioritizing your days to start honing in on what you want, setting yourself up for success. Ask yourself what are the things you really enjoy doing? Baking? Creating art? Helping others? Animals? What are the things you find yourself constantly having to pull yourself away from or, wishing desperately that you had the time to do? Is there a problem you are passionate about solving? Something that is plaguing you in your life that you could fix? The ability to express yourself through how you solve problems can become your passion, as it did for me. And remember that this isn't life or death - it's ok to explore things that you think MIGHT be your passion. If you find at a future date that while you enjoyed pursuing it, but that it didn't turn out to be the final, end all calling that couldn't be ignored just remember that you had fun and that you have still moved yet another step forward. Some people experience multiple passions in their lifetime - several strong drives that can each last for years before being replaced by something equally or, perhaps more strong than the previous pursuit. For others, time is the key to finding their passion. Just as most people don't truly experience love at first sight, finding your passion isn't always like being struck by lighting. Sometimes it's more like an wonderful friendship where strong feelings grow over time into a huge river of deep love.

You might not have all of the tools yourself but, you must find them. You don't have to have all of the answers, you just have to become the kind of person that will find the right people or, sources of information that will allow you to gain the answers. And sometimes you will just need to take a path and see what happens, because the correct direction is not always evident. As long as you continually pay attention to the results, you will be moving forward either way because if you end up selecting the "wrong" path, at least you have eliminated an option and now know not to go that way again.

In my case, I had an early passion for reading and learning about the things that could make me better, healthier, stronger, and a more well rounded athlete. Nutrition and exercise were my first loves in life, and applying it in my very own life and those of others is what drove me, what made me happy, and what made me feel fulfilled. I have helped people lose their baby weight, athletes get stronger, people get leaner to play sports and do things that they couldn't earlier because of their weight, and I helped many women to finally reach such amazing competition shape that they were able to stand on stage in a bikini in front of hundreds of people. What continually amazes me is just how profound the changes are to people's minds and spirits after they focus so hard on disciplining their bodies. In some cases they became totally different people who later become the beacon of light that inspires many others. Some of them also have since found their passions in life due to their transformations.

Even though I knew my passion early in life I still ended up in a position once where I chose a job that was outside the field I loved due to life circumstances. I tried to make the best of it for a while but knew my heart was not in it. I didn't see a way out at the time but I knew that I would never feel fulfilled or, comfortable until I was doing what I was passionate about once again. The creation of Quest Nutrition was my way of going back to my roots and finding a way to create a product that was directly in support of my passion. I now get to work with people on an international level doing what I desire, simply because I refused to settle for a life that was safe but that didn't set my soul on fire.

If you love what you do, you never work a day in your life.

Shannan Yorton Penna

I've been passionate about health and nutrition my whole life. I created Quest Nutrition because I believed that it's possible to have exceptional taste without compromising your nutrition.

VOLUME III - ACHIEVE SUCCESS

The Power of Positive Thinking
by Victoria Adelus

You can do anything you set your mind to. You've probably heard that line more than a million times. Your parents may have preached it to you as a child or maybe your boss repeats it as a reminder in your adult life. It's a timeless saying that couldn't be closer to the truth. Whether or not you believe it's true, you're right.

Your mind has the power to conceive great things. In fact, just about anything you can visualize you can accomplish. However, few allow their thoughts to develop their full potential. Instead, most people to do quite the opposite.

If you embrace the power of positive thinking, new experiences and opportunities will come your way. A positive perspective has the potential to reduce stress, build confidence, and develop character. Practicing how to "look on the bright side" has also proved to fight off the common cold, reduce the risk of death from disease, and enable people to lead healthier lives.

It does, however, take time to develop this perspective, and it's not something that happens overnight. To excel at anything in life, one must work on it daily. Just like you train your body in the gym, you've also got to train your mind. I'm a firm believer that intently developing your body and mind is the only way to successfully reach your goals, no matter the magnitude.

Most people are programed to expect the worst. Many often give up on themselves before they even start. As soon as you allow negativity or doubt to creep in, you're more likely to take a step backward than leap forward toward what you want to achieve. If you think you can't do it, you won't. If you don't think you're strong enough, you probably aren't.

But, if you change that thought process now, you'll be surprised at what you can accomplish.

So where do you start? First, make sure to surround yourself with positive and like-minded people. When I first entered the fitness world I quickly found out who was there for me, and who wasn't. In fact, the friends who I thought had my back ridiculed me for my fitness goals, and people I didn't even know ended up being the ones cheering for me on the sidelines. Identify the negative people in your life. Recognize that they do not add to your mission, and are most likely holding you back. Make a change and associate yourself with people who genuinely want you to be happy and successful. Negative people and thoughts breed negative actions, and that's the last thing you need on your journey toward optimism.

Again, train your mind and your body will follow. Instead of fixating on a negative event that happened during your day, focus on the positive. We as humans tend to turn small dilemmas into catastrophes and blow minor speed bumps out of proportion. Don't allow one negative thought or action take over your entire day, month, or year. Acknowledge it happened, learn from it, and move onward and upward. It's so important to recognize progress, no matter how small. At first, you may even need to write down positive accomplishments or thoughts to make sure you appreciate them and are headed in the right direction. Remember, visualization and positive thoughts take time to develop.

Another way you can build mental strength is by setting a foundation of healthy habits. If you are currently eating food that's bad for you, and you're not exercising, it's going to be very challenging to find an optimistic approach to life. You simply won't feel or look good. Make a commitment to yourself, and put it into action. I promise, taking care of yourself and following your new positive outlook will create a snowball effect throughout all facets of your life. Your positive actions will breed positive thoughts, and those positive thoughts will produce more positive actions. It's been proven time and time again that exercise and eating right can make you feel better, on the inside and out.

Positive thoughts also start with self-respect and the feelings you have toward yourself. If you constantly put yourself down or focus on your flaws, how can you believe that you can achieve anything? Instead of picking yourself apart, give yourself a compliment. Yes, stop reading this for a second and say something nice about yourself. Seriously, put the book down, and do it RIGHT NOW.

See, don't you feel better already? Every time you find yourself thinking or saying negative things about yourself, always come back with a compliment. Loving yourself and developing your strengths will enable you to feel like you can conquer the world.

Remember, it all starts with a single thought, and that one belief can change your life and its direction. Make a plan to practice positive thinking on a daily basis. Some days will be more challenging than others, but that's what makes life so great. Embrace the good with the bad and always shift your focus away from negativity. Visualize each mistake or slip-up as a lesson instead of a failing moment. Only you can create the world you live in, and it really is a choice. Choose wisely, and believe that anything is possible!

> "Watch your thoughts; they become words. Watch your words; they become actions. Watch your actions; they become habit. Watch your habits; they become character. Watch your character; it becomes your destiny." – Lao Tzu

Victoria Adelus

I'm an IFBB Figure Pro, All American EFX and Quest Athlete, Media Personality, Coach, Oddo's Angel and Former NBC Affiliate News Anchor.

5 Steps to Making Your Dreams Come True by Bex Borucki

They often say success comes to those who believe in themselves, but it was the knowledge that I had nothing left to lose that pushed me down what was at first an unforeseeable path. It made it easy to leap and believe the net would some how appear when I was already so low to the ground. This became a devoted daily practice. And out of mere rituals came miracles, and miracles allowed me to believe in myself.

And so now I sit here at 6 AM at the desk in the home office I created. I'm surrounded by my favorite things. They are artifacts on the altar of my life: a framed portrait of Wonder Woman, a light-up statue of the Buddha, a unicorn bust, a tiny pink elephant, my children's artwork, a newspaper article celebrating my business, a photograph of me as a baby sitting on my now-deceased father's lap. Heirlooms of the people and objects that have fed my success.

I feed myself - I've made inspiration boards. I keep stacks of books by friends and people I admire. I place these things in my narrowed personal perspective as a frame of reference to remind myself of the beauty, wisdom, and whimsy the Universe has to offer.

Rituals. Simple, yet undeniably foremost in staying on this journey upward. My gratitude journal also sits in front of me. It peeks at me from behind my laptop screen. This journal is a container of my most precious expressions of love for my life. It's a miracle in paper form. It's my daily teacher and the facilitator for self-knowledge. There are only three spots available on each day's page to list what has brought joy to my day. I've never had a problem filling them in with swift excitement. Even on my heaviest days, when emotional, financial, or physical responsibilities feel too burdensome to bear, I find lightness in the act of picking up a pen to list the three moments that shined brightly on whatever dismay laid before me. Finding light in the dark… yep, that IS the miracle.

Yet, as I sit here upon my meditation cushion in my dark office, I also experience a tiny pang of unease. This is not the future I imagined for myself as a little girl. More pointedly: this is not a future I believed was available to me. I have four beautiful children, a husband who adores me and for whom I adore. We have a warm home surrounded by expansive woods. I have a fit and healthy body, and a career that serves my heart and helps support my family – this is more than I could have asked for and certainly more than I could have fathomed as my life.

How did I get here? Is this really all for me?

Irrational fears are always cropping up. If this life isn't meant for me, then I'll most certainly be found out. It can all be taken from me in an instant – not just my things or my circumstances, but all of the people I love, too. There's this feeling that I'm perpetrating some sort of fraud, that I'm an actor playing a part. The sad little girl who grew up with very little in regard to things or affection, who turned into the adult woman who never demanded (or commanded) love or respect from the people she allowed to get close to her, is now somehow a woman teaching other women how to love themselves and free themselves from the prison of abuse and self-doubt? It makes no sense. Surely, the truth will be revealed and all of my insignificance and ineptitude will become glaringly obvious to everyone.

The reality is that all of those irrational fears are part of a hateful un-reality. They are thoughts meant to keep me from growing and hoping, but they are also thoughts meant to keep me feeling safe. The trouble with fear is that it sometimes brings us comfort. It tricks us into thinking that our circumstances are just as they should be only for the fact that they feel familiar. For me, abuse, neglect, lack of affection, and poverty were all conditions and ideas that I had grown used to in my younger years. As a terrible consequence of my familiarity with lack, abundance felt uncomfortable and suspicious. I resisted those times as a foreign intrusion. I sabotaged my happiness because it felt wrong to be happy.

Today, as a woman who experiences abundance in every aspect of her life, I am constantly managing those old irrational fears of being found out as hoax and losing all that I love. Perhaps it's going to take a time for those fears to disappear completely.

However, at one time they were a constant agitator that plagued my thoughts and body with anxiety, now they are just cautionary pangs of discomfort here and there that show up when anything really good happens.

I still ask myself "How did I get here?" But I do so on more positive and curious terms. How did I manage to create this life, despite all the fear, doubt, and lack of self-love that for a lifetime felt imbued in the fabric of my existence? The simple and true answer is that I made it my personal everyday practice to act in spite of my fear. I was afraid, but I did it anyway. I would literally ask myself, "What's the worst that could happen?" before every business call, before I clicked the publish button on every blog, and before every yoga class where dozens of eyes would be staring at me, waiting for me to begin teaching. As silly as it sounds, knowing that I wouldn't die, that my kids couldn't be taken from me, or that I wouldn't end up homeless as a result of a singular mess-up made me feel ok with taking the leap and risking total humiliation. Almost, it's a journey.

The act of believing in myself did not breed my success. The knowledge that I had nothing more to lose freed up the space towards success and allowed the net to appear. Then miracles started to appear and I started believing in myself. The doubt started to fade away and give way to the synchronistic events that led to my success. It's a daily practice.

Every once in a while, I write down a short of list of ways to achieve success. I use the word success to describe a myriad of states of being. Success can come in the form of satisfaction with your job, happiness in your relationships, pride in your accomplishments, and so on. There are times when I feel so successful, my heart feels like it may burst. There are mornings when I wake up with such gratitude, excitement, and curiosity for what the day ahead may hold in store for me that I find it impossible to stay in bed for another moment. A little more than a year ago, I wrote another one of my short lists to outline some methods I've used for finding personal success in the form of dreams coming true, and I posted it on my blog. I want to re-share a revised version with you today:

Step 1 – Believe in dreams and miracles. Have a dream, and believe that it can come true.

That's it. Believe that dreams and miracles happen every day. You also have to acknowledge that you've already experienced countless big and tiny miracles in your own life. The fact that I'm able to communicate with people all over the world every single day through a marvelous machine of modern science and technology through an interconnected invisible network called the internet is kind of miraculous. Bam! There's a miracle. Every "I want…" is a little dream. Kaplow! You already have your first dream.

Step 2 – Speak your dreams OUT LOUD.

Bring your dreams out of your imagination and into reality with your breath and your words. Tell everyone you meet about all the amazing things that are coming your way. Speak it, and you'll start to believe it. You'll also be planting tiny little promises all around that you're just going to have to fulfill. Sometimes speaking a dream out loud can be the scariest thing imaginable. "What will people think of me? Will they find me egotistical or too proud or obnoxious?" Who cares! Your desire for happiness is so valid and so worth fighting for. Maybe you think you don't deserve it right now or that it's not for you. That cannot matter. Just keep talking about your dreams, wants, and desires as if you already have them – as if they're already on their way. Then watch closely for what happens next.

Step 3 – Show up.

When people start hearing about your dreams, they'll want to be a part of them. They'll think of you when something in their own life pops up that reminds them of your dream. They'll tell you about opportunities and want to connect you with people who share your passion. There is a catch. You have to be ready to show up for these opportunities – even if you're impossibly afraid. Fear will try to get in your way at every turn. Just thank this fear for its time and contribution to your growing process, and then move right past it. Show up even when you're not quite sure what you're doing. Show up even when you're not sure if you'll get anything out of the experience. Just keep showing up every single day. Don't make it hard for your dreams to find you. By the way, "show up" also means "work really bloody hard" on your passion. Dreams always require hard work.

Step 4 – Be kind and be grateful.

I can say a lot about why this is probably the most important step, but I'll keep it simple. Just practice kindness and gratitude, and the Universe (and your friends and family and strangers) will reward you with even more to be grateful for and relationships to practice your newfound appreciation and benevolence. Be kind to people who reflect who you may have been. Show compassion for them and offer your help and guidance in order to lift them up with you. Share your knowledge, your success stories, and truth about your missteps and failures. Always offer your most authentic self, because that's all that the Universe wants from you. Acknowledge how much you have to be grateful for, and be grateful that you have so much to offer.

Step 5 – Save for a rainy (or sunny) day.

This applies to money, energy, ideas and time. You can't give everything to everything. Make it your practice to focus on one thing at this very moment. Practice being here now. It's important to save a little back for the big miracles that pop up out of nowhere and need a little extra "something" to make them work. Even joy can overwhelm you. Great opportunities can cause you to shut down. Approach your everyday life with softness and save your energy for the times that require hard work.

There will always be times when great tragedy presents itself to you. If you use up too much energy worrying about your laundry pile, your stack of bills, or what your co-worker thinks of you, your power will be too depleted to carry you through that pain or sadness.

My father died recently. At the time of his death I was experiencing unprecedented success in my life. Beyond personal successes, my professional life was moving stealthily toward abundance. He watched the first episode of my first television show on his deathbed just days before he passed. We watched together with excitement and pride.

If my practice wasn't to focus on gratitude every single day, I would have missed all the beauty of being with him during his final days and hours. I would have only felt the sadness. It's a miracle to have a practice.

Success, satisfaction, self-love, dream building - these all take practice and disciplined work. The greater practice is to remind yourself on a constant basis that all of these things are absolutely for you. The act of reminding continues to be my practice. Fear creeps in, and I act in spite of it. Doubt takes hold, and I breathe deeply until it lets go. Rules are presented to me, and I write my own instead. My greatest wish is for you to do the same… or better. I love you!

Bex Borucki

I'm the founder of BEXLIFE™ and the BLISSED IN™ wellness movement. A blissfully married mother-of-four, TV host, fitness and yoga instructor, popular YouTuber, and backyard farmer raising chickens and goats.

The Fitness Journey of Kelsey Byers
by Kelsey Byers

I love sharing my weight loss story because many people I meet are struggling to achieve their own fitness and wellness goals. I have been told that my story gives people hope and helps them set realistic goals for themselves. I lost fifty pounds after college and I'm in the best shape of my life at age thirty-one. One day I looked in the mirror and realized I was fed up with feeling bad about myself. It all started with a decision to change my lifestyle. The rest is history.

My story

I was very active in high school. Growing up in a small town, I was able to play all sports. I could eat like a pig and still be a string bean. I played basketball, volleyball, golf, track, cross-country and was on our school dance team. Once I got to college, my activity level decreased significantly. I also adopted some bad habits like drinking alcohol, staying out late and eating fast food.

The weight "snuck up" on me. I am a tall woman, 5'10 to be exact. I graduated high school weighing 130 - 135 pounds. At my heaviest weight in college, I weighed almost 180 pounds. I could not believe I had put on about fifty pounds in a matter of only two years. The weight came on so quickly that I had sizes ranging from four to fourteen in my closet. I was not happy with my body and I actually went shopping all the time, always looking for that perfect outfit to make my body look better. It never happened. The day it all hit me was a HUGE reality check. I overheard someone refer to me as a "whale." It really hit home because this was someone I knew personally and I had been thin my entire life. This was the first time I struggled with weight.

I was not happy with the person I saw in the mirror and I knew I needed a lifestyle change. I was never one for dieting and got bored quickly with salads. I finally realized that when you have a great body, everything looks great on you. Once I was honest with myself and mapped out my goals, I started making small changes here and there. I started going out to eat less and committed myself to working out two or three days a week. It took me five years of trial and error to get rid of most of the weight. I later found out I could have dropped the weight in just a matter of months if I had only understood how big a role nutrition plays in how you look and feel.

I dropped from a size fourteen to an eight and felt really healthy for the first time in years. I took more of an interest in fitness and decided to challenge myself even more in the gym and aimed at sculpting a lean body. That's when I heard about clean eating. My definition of clean eating is consuming non-processed meals every three hours, five to seven meals a day. I hired a nutritionist in March 2010 and my body drastically changed within just three months of consistent clean eating.

Who would have thought I needed to eat more to lose weight and get lean? My meal plan consists of 1,800-2,000 healthy calories a day. Since I eat every three hours, I always feel satisfied with my meals and it cuts down on cravings. I don't obsess with weighing myself or counting calories on a daily basis. My husband and I cook in bulk two days a week. We save money each month by avoiding restaurants and save going out to eat for special occasions.

I know what foods work for my body and I plan a cheat meal every week or two to indulge. You have to find that perfect balance for your mind and body. I have found that by eating clean year round, I never have to "diet" or struggle with my weight. It's the best feeling in the world. I believe that nutrition determines 80% of how you look, exercise being

20%. This explains why I spent years in the gym but did not get the results I was after until I focused on nutrition.

I make small weekly goals to stay on track and hold myself accountable. I lift weights three to four days per week and include thirty minutes of cardio three days a week. It is not necessary to work out for hours each day. In fact, it's very easy to over train your body, especially when your nutrition is not on point.

Since my journey with eating clean, I have set several big goals for myself and am very proud to say that I have accomplished each one. These include writing my first book in order to help others, compete in fitness competitions, becoming a spokes model for one of the top nutrition companies in the industry, appearing on the cover of Oxygen Magazine and more. You can accomplish your goals; just go at it with everything you have. Take small steps each week that all lead to the big goal at the end. Hold yourself accountable.

"Begin to think of yourself as they person you want to be."
"Eat clean and follow your dreams."

Thank you for your interest in my story,

Kelsey Byers
I'm a mommy-to-be, author, fitness blogger, model, Labrada Nutrition sponsored athlete, graduate student. 50-pound weight loss story. I love helping others.

The Power of Choice
by Jacqueline Carly

I officially started dieting when I was eight years old. Before that I had dabbled in skipping some meals here and there, and doing leg lifts in my room, but I hadn't really committed to a plan. Weight Watcher meetings were every Monday night. There was a weigh-in in front of the group, then a check-in and meeting. My best friend and I were the only kids there. I remember being told I should drink a lot of iced water throughout the day, because it burned calories. All it did for me was always make me shiver.

By the time I was in high school I was 180lbs and had tried the hot dog and waffle diet, the hamburger meat and water diet, the cabbage soup diet, the banana diet, the grapefruit diet, the vinegar and egg diet, and the list goes on and on. Remember Deal-a-meal? Yeah, that one too. There was no end for the hatred I felt for my body, and I would do whatever it took to make it do what I wanted.

Enter bulimia and clinical depression into my life.

What seemed like a cool and easy way to eat whatever I wanted, while not gaining weight, quickly turned into an obsession and addiction. My entire world soon revolved around binging and purging, exercising, and taking laxatives and amphetamines. I'd call in sick to work and break off plans with friends just so I could stay home and binge. There was no room for anything else in my life for the next seven years.

I'd like to say that I woke up one day, turned my life around and all was well, but it didn't happen that way. What followed was a long, winding journey full of stumbles and falls. It would be a while before the part of me that wanted to get well was greater than the part that did not.

Have you ever felt that way? You want to make a change, but you feel so stuck and overwhelmed it's seems easier to give up? I've felt it many times. But as I've learned, it's always only temporary.

As you've probably already guessed, I did eventually get well. Otherwise, I wouldn't have the privilege of sharing my story with you here. But my story is not unique. My story is your story and your story is my story. Our circumstances, struggles, pains, or fears might be different, but you and I both have the power within us to make a different choice. We can choose ourselves. We can choose to be whoever we want to be.

Who do you want to be? What goals do you have? What's your BIG dream? Seriously, I want to know! Send me an email and share your dream: Fitarella@gmail.com.

I've sat with that question many times over the years, and it's changed a quite a few times as I've evolved. However, the one thing that has never changed is the commitment I made to myself many years ago, to devote myself to spreading LOVE and helping people shine their brightest light.

And that is what I want for you.

I want you to blaze like the sun and rock your life!

I've spent the last 15 years dedicated to studying the inner and outer workings of the body. I've earned my Masters in Nutrition, am completing my PhD in MindBody Medicine, and have a myriad of certifications in fitness, yoga, crossfit, and endurance training. What I know for sure is that, we are all connected and the mind, body, & spirit are one. We are whole beings that need to love and be loved, and we need to be nurtured and well fed. Not just our bellies, but our mind and spirit, too.

Take a moment to think about how you feed yourself. Do you surround yourself with positive people that support you? Do you spend time doing the things you love? Do you move your body every day, fuel it whole foods and treat it with respect? Do you exercise your mind and broaden your horizons?

What do you need more of in your life?

Only you know what you need, and only you are responsible for making sure you get it. You're not much use to yourself or anyone else, if you're not at your best. Treating yourself with love, kindness and respect is the foundation upon which everything else is built. So, what's one thing that's missing from your self-care that you can begin to give yourself every week?

Whatever it is, give yourself this gift and commit to it right now.

Earlier I asked you about your big dream and about who you want to be. Do you have answers to those questions? Before you can begin anything, you have to get clear on what it is you REALLY want. Do you want to go to school? Lose weight? Change careers? Travel the world? Start a business? If you're thinking yes to all of the above that's ok, but start with one goal. I spent many fine years being a jack-of- all-trades and master of none, but when I wanted to take my success to the next level I had to work on one thing at a time to give it the full attention it deserved. Having clarity on what your final destination is will help keep you focused during the journey, and act as a filter to weed out what doesn't serve you.

After you've chosen your goal, write it down and post it everywhere. Put it in your agenda, on the refrigerator, on your calendar, in your office, keep a copy in your purse, etc. The more you see it and are reminded of what you're working toward, the more it will light your fire and inspire to keep going.

Two years ago for my birthday, I wanted the word patience tattooed on my right wrist, and practice tattooed on my left. These words have deep meaning for me, and having them tattooed would be a constant reminder of, what I feel are, important lessons on my journey. Before getting the tattoos, I searched hi and low for the right tattoo artist to ensure they would come out perfect. I was down to three artists, but it turned out they were all booked for months. MONTHS! But I couldn't wait for months, I wanted them NOW or else my birthday would be ruined. So, I settled and randomly chose a local place, rationalizing that they were only words, how could anyone screw it up?

Well, guess what? They got screwed up.

Ah yes, the irony of getting the words patience & practice tattooed on myself, while not being patient enough to wait, and not ending up with what I wanted, is definitely not lost on me. A cosmic joke, for sure! However, after the dust settled (and after a lot of tears later) I chose to shift my perspective and see the situation in a different light. The words on my wrist would still continue to be a reminder of my work with patience and practice, but now they would also serve as a reminder of the beauty of imperfection.

How we chose to see things determines our experience. What things "mean" to us, determines our experience.

Tony Robbins said "What you link pain to, and what you link pleasure to shape your destiny.".

On the path to your goal you will undoubtedly encounter obstacles, because nothing worth getting is easy. But that doesn't mean you're not supposed to have it, or that you're not good enough. Or that you don't have what it takes. All it means is that there's work to be done. That's it. And I believe, from the bottom of my heart, that you can do it.

This book is filled with stories of women that have overcome adversity to live their dreams, and you are no different.

YOU are in the driver's seat, and no matter what, you always have a choice. You have everything you need inside of you and your dream is worth it.

YOU ARE WORTH IT!

Miriam Khalladi

The world needs your gifts; don't keep it waiting any longer. Choose yourself, right now.

> "Always seek less turbulent skies. Hurt. Fly above it.
> Betrayal. Fly above it.
> Anger. Fly above it.
> You are the one who is flying the plane."
> - Marianne Williamson

Jacqueline Carly

I'm a mom, MindBody Medicine Scientist, athlete and entrepreneur fiercely devoted to helping people feel better in their bodies and love themselves more.

Finding My Delicious Passion
by Tess Challis

It seems like just yesterday that I was standing outside the restaurant I waitressed at, wondering if I'd ever find my passion. I was a college graduate who had majored in art and philosophy (two fields that are barely relevant to the work I do now) and working at a job that left me very little time to think about what I wanted to do with my life. I had skills in several areas: jewelry making; singing and playing guitar; painting; designing; cooking; and yes - waiting tables! However, being a "jack of all trades," I'd always found it hard to zero in on just one thing.

Years passed and after I'd worked at an assortment of random jobs (interior design, cleaning houses, and selling furniture), I found myself admitting that I wasn't living my passion. Incidentally, at this point I'd been vegan for about 15 years and had built up a large repertoire of delicious plant-based recipes. For me, cooking for people and "turning them on" to vegan food was sheer ecstasy! Nothing thrilled me more than feeding someone wild mushroom lasagna or chocolate pie and hearing them say "Wow, I can't believe this is vegan! This is the most delicious thing I've ever eaten!"

The very first time I'd heard those words was around 1992. I'd originally gone on a plant-based diet in 1991 for reasons unrelated to health. However, what I noticed within a mere two weeks on my new "diet" blew me away - my embarrassing acne cleared up, I was no longer anemic, I finally had energy, and I stopped getting constant bouts of strep throat and other illnesses. However, there was still a slight problem - as a lover of good food, I was worried! Back then, there were no reliable vegan cookbooks on the market and the restaurant scene was dismal. As someone who enjoyed food a bit too much, I knew I'd never stick with any sort of healthy lifestyle unless it could be enjoyable for me. So, for the next year, I cooked my hungry little butt off, trying to come up with reliable recipes that were truly satisfying to me. There were far more failures than successes at first, but I didn't give up. Any time I made a dish that was delicious - especially one that my friends and family raved about - was a tiny victory.

For years, I continued working at a variety of jobs and cooking in my spare time. The first time I did anything remotely career-wise was in 1997 when I began teaching my co-workers how to make smoothies. I'd bring my blender to the furniture store and we'd all make healthy smoothies on our break! Soon after, a few of the ladies I worked with asked me to hold a cooking class. I was so excited! I had them over to my house and showed them how to make creamy blintzes, asparagus linguine, chocolate dream pie, and Florentine bread salad. They loved it!

I continued on for the next year, holding classes occasionally, until I decided to quit my day job and be a full time personal chef and caterer. This was great for a while - I had some wonderful clients. However, after a year or two I found that cooking for others left me exhausted and depleted. It was not my passion. I much preferred the excitement of showing others how to cook. I wanted to put the power in their hands.

It was several years later that I finally listened to the many people who had strongly suggested I write a cookbook. I'd brushed the idea off for years, thinking it would be too much work. However, I couldn't ignore the requests any longer, and finally decided to do it. Besides, it would probably only take about two weeks, right? How hard could it be? Two years later, after countless edits and a steep learning curve, my first book was finally done. I sat there, book in hand, thinking "I will never do this again!" It felt like I'd just had a baby! But unlike some babies who let their mothers sleep through the night (my actual baby didn't do that either, but that's another story), a book needs constant tending. I'd been under some sort of illusion that all I had to do was write the book, and somehow I'd end up on the NY Times bestseller list. Yet another learning experience was born - I now had to master the crafts of social media, updating my website, and blogging. It was a lot of work, and especially after finding myself without a day job again, it was often scary. I loved creating recipes and inspiring others to eat better, but I wasn't sure I could pull it off as a career - in fact, I really doubted I could. Money was tight and I was a single mother, doing everything on a shoestring budget.

However, an interesting thing started to happen. People began to tell me things that made it impossible to stop. I'd get an email that said "Thanks to your book, my whole family is eating better" or "Thanks to you, my mom no longer has cancer." I've gotten emails from people telling me everything from "You've helped me overcome an eating disorder" to "This is the only way I've ever been able to lose weight without feeling deprived." Emails even came from people just wanting to tell me that they appreciated having delicious recipes they could count on - ones that made it easy to eat a healthy plant-based diet. It was exhilarating! I finally felt I was doing what I'd been meant to do. Not only did I enjoy creating delicious, healthy recipes, but I'd found something I loved even more - empowering people to eat better and live better. It was, and is, truly joyful!

Years later, I'm still happily immersed in the same field - I've now written four books and added wellness coaching to my repertoire. It's not always easy, but it's always worth it. At this point, there have been countless emails, letters, and testimonials from people who've thanked me for writing those books, or for being their coach.

If I ever get tired and wonder if I can keep doing what I'm doing, those are the things that immediately recharge me and keep me going. We all have a gift to share, and I'm so thankful I've found mine. Truly, nothing can be more joyful than doing what you love and being able to empower others in the process!

I'd like to share what I feel are the Five Steps to Finding Your Passion. I hope you find them inspiring and helpful - and I wish you joy on your journey to finding your passion and living with purpose!

1. Go Where the Energy Flows: This is a woo-woo way of saying it's possible to sense what is and isn't on your path. Can you remember a time when something (a job or relationship, for example) was no longer working? The energy felt "dead" to you. On the other hand, have you ever been drawn to something? There is "alive" energy there for you. Explore that. Go where the energy is flowing, and let go of what no longer holds energy for you.

2. Be Open to Change: Just because you began a certain path doesn't mean you need to continue on it forever! We often need to have a variety of experiences as stepping stones to find what we're ultimately destined for.

3. Choose Love: Whenever we're faced with a tough decision, we can boil our options down to two things - love or fear. It's easy to make decisions based on fear, but when we trust and follow where love leads, things work out beautifully. I've often followed the Zen saying "Leap and the net will appear." People have called me foolish, but it has always, always worked out.

4. Experiment! Give yourself the opportunity to explore the things that call to you. If you've always wondered what pottery would be like, take a class! Play and have fun. Try new things. It's when we allow ourselves to follow our bliss that we find our passion.

5. Don't Give Up: When you do find your passion, please know how important persistence is. Things often take a lot of work and time. Just because you've been told "no" by ten publishers does not mean you should

give up writing! On the contrary. Do you know that the Beatles were told they'd never make it as musicians? That Oprah was told she wasn't a good fit for TV? Don't listen to the critics - persist, don't give up, and put in your time. The only way to fail is to give up!

Tess Challis
I'm an author, vegan chef and wellness coach.

Failure - The Greatest Secret to Success by Diana Chaloux-LaCerte

If you look closely at the life patterns of highly successful individuals, you will find a common, recurring theme. Whether you study the lives of those who have achieved major milestones in business, in their career or finances, or physically and within a certain industry such as the world of fitness, these superstars may come from a wide variety of backgrounds, ethnicities and income levels, but regardless of origin, you will discover that they have all, to one degree or another, experienced something powerful in their lives that has aided in their catapult to the top of the food chain. That something is Failure.

Sounds a little crazy right? If these people are so successful, it should mean that they've lived a charmed life, always made good choices and never had to experience the pain of falling flat on their face, losing a battle that they intensely wanted to win, or made down-right bad decisions that led to drawbacks financially, physically, emotionally, spiritually or in personal relationships? Right?

On the contrary! Successful people are usually the ones who at one point or another have failed miserably, have taken giant leaps of faith only to find their wings are not yet fastened securely and they come crashing to the ground. In the world of finance, the greatest successes are typically those who have at one point been bankrupt or had business failures. In career, many who have achieved the highest levels of success in any industry have had multiple doors slammed in their faces, heard the word "No" repeatedly and been rejected on many occasions. In the world of fitness, many of the top faces and leading names that you see have experienced failure on different levels. Perhaps they were at one point failing in the area of physical healthy, countless top models today have stories of at one point being overweight, unhealthy and unhappy in their lives. Or perhaps they have competed and didn't place where they wanted to, or were denied or rejected an opportunity that they truly wanted.

What is it about failure that leads these people to even greater achievement? If this is a common theme in the successful, how come every person who has failed in their life, isn't reaching these higher echelons of success?

The power of failure is all in the way that you view it, and where you choose to put your focus in the aftermath of a perceived failure.

The people who look at themselves, something in their life, or the outcome of a certain event as a failure, and process that information as meaning that they are useless, not good enough, or not competent enough to pursue their goal, are the ones who are going to quit moving forward, curl up in a little ball of fear and stop making progress towards their goals. These are the people who will remain status quo or less, they will stick with pathways that they feel are safe and have low risk of feeling that pain of failure again, these are people that will never attain a high level of success.

On the other hand, there is a different way that failure can be viewed. A powerful and productive perspective that can get you so fired up, so determined, that you become unstoppable! Failure is nothing more than feedback, information that you can use to make better or different choices in the future. With every failure you have the opportunity to learn and grow. You have a chance to make improvements, change your course of action, and try again or take an alternate route, and you now have the advantage of a higher level of knowledge and a higher level of experience. The next time you make a choice or take a chance in any facet of your life, you are going to have a higher chance of succeeding with that failure under your belt.

Your personal definition of failure is important too, this is something you need to be clear about. If you interpret minor setbacks or obstacles (or in the world of fitness for example, not placing exactly where you want to in a competition) as an epic failure, then you are setting yourself up for a world of unnecessary high levels of pain and upset. Those who end up being ultimately successful at aspects in their lives are able to understand levels of failure and assign an appropriate level of importance to them. Looking at every little bump in the road as a major disaster isn't going to be productive in the long run, but rather lead to feelings of resentment, guilt, inadequacy and depression. These are negative emotions that aren't going to fuel you in the right direction.

When you have, what you consider in your mind, failed at something, what are some of the emotions that you feel? Identifying these emotions is one way that you can recognize the opportunity for growth and improvement. Here are a couple of the most common.

First is disappointment. It's of course a natural human response to failure. But it is something you must be careful with. You can use disappointment in a negative way and decide that you should just not go after your goal any longer, OR you can change your perspective. Are there any positives that you took away from the situation? Did you learn anything from the situation that will allow you to improve or find an alternate route to the goal? Does the failure mean that a door is entirely closed or if you look around could there be a new window that has opened up?

Another common emotion is frustration. This is actually a great emotion to have. When you feel frustrated, that means that you feel that you should have or could have achieved a goal, it bothers you that you didn't. This powerful emotion can lead you to going back to the drawing board, convinced that you CAN achieve what you want, and develop a new strategy for getting where you ultimately want to be.

Don't play the blame game. When you have failed at something, even if you may have every right to point the finger of blame on a person or situation, this isn't going to lead to productivity, even if in your mind it is completely the truth of the situation. And guess what, you may be 100% right! But placing blame on anyone or anything else for failure is ultimately giving the power of the situation and the future of your success, to the person or event. To be the most successful, you don't want to give that power away, YOU want to have that power at all times, because ultimately it is YOU who are going to be the reason you are a success.

Fear of failure is paralyzing. It is the one thing that will keep you grounded exactly where you are in life. It can prevent you from ever taking major strides towards goals and dreams that you wish you could attain.

If you want something in life, you have to overcome your fear of failure and go for it. Whether your goal is to own your own business, be a multi millionaire, find an amazing relationship, step on stage for your first time or become a top fitness athlete, if you are afraid to take the action necessary to get to your goals, and if you're afraid that at some point you are going to be rejected or fail or make a bad decision, then the one thing I can promise is that you will never get where you want to be! Chances are that you ARE going to "fail" at something, you are going to be disappointed or frustrated, you may very well be rejected on certain occasions, and there is very high likelihood that you will make stupid mistakes throughout your journey. But you know what? That is ok! You want to make mistakes and you want to fail!

I do consider myself a successful person, that doesn't mean I'm at the ultimate level of success that I ultimately want to be, but for the place in life that I'm currently at, I am happy with many of the things I've achieved on multiple levels of life, including physical, mental, spiritual, financial and relationship wise. I'm such a strong believer in the power of failure and it is because I've personally failed in every single one of these areas that I now feel successful in, at one point or another. I failed physically when I let myself get 40 pounds overweight in my mid twenties, I let the pain of that failure fuel me to want to compete. I've had multiple failed relationships, but discovered more about myself through each one and ultimately that has allowed me to find a relationship with my husband that surpasses even what my greatest expectations could have been. I've failed in business… miserably… I started a company, invested loads of money and my families money only to have the entire thing crash and burn. Miserable is actually not even a strong enough word to describe that failure. But I learned so much from all the mistakes that were made, that it prepared me to make much wiser choices in my business now! When it comes to the world of competition, I've had some great success for sure, but that didn't come without "failure" too. I've lost close competitions and have even been on stages where I went completely unnoticed. I definitely felt the sting of defeat, and the pain of frustration, but ultimately, decided to view every experience as a positive, as a stepping stone and as an opportunity for growth towards doing better the next time or finding something that was a better fit for my ultimate personal goals. I know I'm not done learning, and I know I'm going to make more mistakes and fail many more times in areas of life. But I'm not afraid, I'm excited, because it means getting stronger and better and ultimately it will mean fulfilling the vision of success that I have for myself. That's pretty exciting if you ask me!

To be the most powerful human being you can be, the most successful, the most fulfilled, I encourage you to FAIL FEARLESSLY. Learn from every opportunity and use all of the knowledge and feedback you get to form yourself into the greatest success you can possibly be.

Real Talk Real Women

Diana Chaloux-LaCerte

I'm a Hitch Fit co-owner, transformation trainer and WBFF pro diva fitness model.

Soul Awakening
by Rosie Chee

Sometimes it takes drastic measures for us to become AWARE of our soul, to ACKNOWLEDGE it, the dreams and desires hidden there, away from not just the world but ourselves because we were not yet ready to accept them. It takes someone special, the most extreme of love and loss, to bring those dreams and desires to the surface, to cause us to turn and look INSIDE ourselves to see what else we keep locked away in the dark. It takes time and it is not easy, looking into your own soul, even if you know how dark it is, despite the light you can radiate in certain presence.

Those drastic measures may have rendered your soul in half, so invested was it, even if you at first did not know why, because for the first time someone else UNDERSTOOD you, SAW you, for who you truly ARE, not accepting that what the world saw was the reality. Someone was there for you, encouraging you, BELIEVING in you, parts of you that had lain dead a lifetime suddenly brimming with hope and the gentle spark of life. You experienced immeasurable joy, eyes bright and faith a guiding light, believing in the beautiful promises sent through time and space, and for the first time, allowed yourself to dream such a dream.

And then suddenly the world went dark and the dream came crashing down in darkness, leaving you lost and confused and full of despair so deep it ached in the deepest depths of your soul, and you cried inside, the tears a seeming never-ending avalanche that threatened to consume you, while outside you smiled and everyone thought your life was so charmed, the rare few who you had let glimpse your soul seeing the torture you lived in, the broken mess, and watched you almost plunge from life itself. In that dark you awakened ANOTHER part of your soul, where you made the truth transparent so that not even you could deny what it was, facing yourself head on as you grasped the full reality of the potential that could become.

From the dark rose a soul that had awakened and EMBRACED both the light and the dark nature of the beauty and the beast. From it stepped forth a WARRIOR determined never to let themselves be vulnerable again to such destruction, albeit more open in their soul than they had ever been, thanks to the touching of that other soul on theirs. It was a soul tempered by more than life itself, for the ultimate experience of the giving of one's soul into the keeping of another, allowing themselves to fully trust one besides themselves, took far greater courage than would ever be known, and in the aftermath, not a risk that soul was ever willing or intended to take again.

But in the ashes of the dream you thought burnt forever, there must have been something left BEHIND, hidden away from even you, a desire that had been awakened from dormant sleep, and even in such despair still clung to the minute threads of hope that even just being alive it might somehow survive, although not yet sure why, since that soul had finally found in it the ability to let GO of the dream that it once held so precious and dear, knowing that sometimes dreams are not meant to be anything more, arguing against it because it believes no dream in our heart is given withOUT reason, but not understanding how it could possibly be fulfilled in the wake of all that had transpired.

And then the unexpected discovery of life in this soul, a light spread from the inside out, taking it unawares, but creating such an AWARENESS, identifying with surprise the cause and seeing the effect, not wanting to believe that such a thing was still possible, or even for it, but coming slowly to understand the seasons that had passed had only prepared it for what was to come. New life came with hope reignited in the soul that was more aware than ever of itself and of others, fully embracing the complexity and wonder, a heart thought forever closed slowly unfurling like a rosebud in the winter frost, to welcome the light of the dawn seeking to warm it.

A soul truly AWAKENED through love, loss, and pain, understanding where it has been, where it is now, and where it must go, no longer fighting the dreams and desires tugged from the depths where they hid for so long, allowing light to filter through the darkness and slowly push it away, accepting and embracing the change, knowing that anything is possible for the one who believes and holds tight to their faith, completely coming "into its own" as it BLOSSOMS before the world, is a wonderful and beautiful thing, one of life's miracles.

Rosie Chee
I'm passionate about helping others think like a champion, train like a warrior and live with a purpose. Faith + Fitness = Lifestyle!

Creating Your Own Future
by Joanne Lee Cornish

I stared at the world map on the wall of my office, a moment that turned my life around forever and yet a moment unnoticed by my co workers close by.

"Is this it?"

"Is this really it?!"

I'm 26 years old, I have a really good job, I make my own hours, have a company home, company car, expense account and a pension fund and I'm looking at the map of the world and the city in which I live is too small to even be acknowledged.

I had just put the phone down on the boyfriend I couldn't shake and as I stare at the map I'm thinking that this one person who lives in this one city that isn't even big enough to show up on the map of the world is dictating my life. The whole world is out there and I'm being led by the nose by the comfort of my life.

"Is this is really it?!"

My name is Joanne Lee Cornish and I first stepped on stage as a bodybuilder when I was 18 years old, back in the 80's when the sport was new and shiny and pretty unheard of.

I had ran track as a teenager and was encouraged to build my legs to help with my speed work and so I joined a gym. That was the first door I opened that would change my life forever. The gym was owned by an Olympian judge named Bill Boyd and within 6 months he had me onstage in a local bodybuilding show. I hope never to come across any photographs from that show but I did win it and so my competitive chapter began.

Winning feels really good, it's a feeling that you are happy to repeat and I was winning a lot. I was always getting ready for the next show, the next diet, the next appearance. The ultimate goal was to win the British Overall Championships and turn professional.

As well as competing I was studying for my Business Degree and by the age of 25 I had won the World Championships and the European Championships, I had my Business Degree, secured an amazing job and at long last I had won the overall British Championships and had my pro card.

"Is this it?!"

Since being a teenager I had always been aiming for the next show or the next exam, now I find myself at the top of a couple of ladders with nothing of great certainty on the horizon. Was I really meant to cruise in this humdrum life where there is no real reason to leave but no real passion to stay.

I had achieved the generation before me's nirvana – the secure corporate job where you marry someone somehow and work until they give you a nice gold watch and the rewards of the pension you have paid into for decades. I couldn't shake it, I was now 26 and this was really it! The lull of life where years slip by until they surprise you with that gold watch and walk you out of the office. This was my life? Really?

A seed had already been planted a couple of months before my map epiphany, a seed that started me doubting this nirvana of corporate happy ever after. I worked for British Steel, I was a steel inspector with clients all over the North West of England, there was a gentleman named Rex who did the same job but with a different territory, he had been with British Steel fifty years. The job involved a lot of driving and we had rather nice company cars which we maintained ourselves and billed the company for the expense.

Rex had been with British Steel since he was 16 years old, now at

66 with the British economy taking a nosedive he had been asked to retire. When it came to his final day at the office, there was no gold watch, no party the company paid for, just a bill for the tires he had put on the company car which were no longer going to be used for company business. After 50 years he got a bill for tires!!

My parents generation had the very real dream of corporate security, get with a great company, give your life to that company and you would always be well taken care of. Rex was a huge wake up call to me – the dream, which had been real for many decades, was no longer real, you create your own future, no one is going to do that for you.

I look again at the map; Rex's desk in the next office is empty. My life is pretty good, I have all I could wish for and I'm only 26 but is this really it?!

I stare at the map some more pondering where is the farthest I can go on this planet, the most distance I can create between this place and another, thankfully this turns out to be Australia. Within a few months I am boarding a plane with a working visa and heading to Oz.

I gave up on the 'dream' and decided to create my own.

That year went by very very fast and soon I had another ticket in hand, this was a ticket back to England. It was November and I was leaving summer in Australia to go back to Winter in England. I didn't have a job to return to, I had no money, no car. It's a long flight from Australia to England and there has to be a stop for the plane to refuel, thankfully (again) the stop was in California. With some cash in my pocket a backpack on my back and a couple of cocktails in my stomach I decide not to take the last leg back to England and I find myself In Los Angeles.

It might seem that I am extremely driven and a bit of a risk taker, that really is not the case. I'm more likely to save money than over spend and I'll lose sleep over debt but the one thing that motivates me more than anything is happiness – I simply cannot stay in a situation where I am not happy.

Age 28 and I'm in Gold's Gym, Venice CA, the most famous gym in the world. I had friends who had vacationed to America just to train in this gym. I'm a Professional Bodybuilder and I couldn't be more at home, I'm rubbing shoulders with the people I had only seen in magazines and I am on a first name basis with movie stars.

My Business Degree was not about to help me now and the one thing I knew and the one thing I loved has always been training. Training and Nutrition is all I ever wanted to read about or study, to take certifications and courses was fun for me and so I started to build my Personal Training Business.

I'm trying to build a business alongside some of the best trainers in the world and maybe it would have been smarter to go to a smaller gym/pond but I stuck it out at the Mecca, I studied more, learnt from others, led by example and so my business grew.

I was competing and jumping through hoops with an attorney I couldn't afford to get my green card through my Professional status. I went from a $500 car to a floor to a second hand futon to my own apartment by the beach.

I made it to the Ms. Olympia stage twice and this really represented my bodybuilding summit, I was happy to put that goal aside and concentrate on the progress of others. 9 years after arriving in America I became a resident, I did it on my own merits of which I am very proud. Now in my 20th year running my own Personal Training and Nutrition business I truly feel I am successful.

I work long hours and yet I don't feel like I have had a job since I was 26.

I haven't had a vacation of more than a week in 20 years and yet I live in Malibu and seldom feel the desire to leave.

I spend every hour of 'work' with a different friend and I work alongside a family of other trainers in a gym that I love as much as the first day I trained there.

There have been ups and downs and feasts and famines and I am happy, incredibly happy.

What I would ask you to take from this tale is that you don't have to be the smartest, the most driven, the most ambitious, the most fearless. Just do not settle for less than you are capable of, do not take the safe road just because the other road looks too rocky and if you are good at something, keep doing it, keep practicing it, keep educating yourself and just keep doing it, do not stop for a second, do not give up when times get hard - if you know you're good and you love doing something just keep doing it, you will succeed.

I would be amiss if I did not acknowledge a few people that made my life possible. I have the most incredible family, I always knew if the bottom fell out of my world I could always go home and I married the most amazing man, nothing makes sense without Kevin.

P.S. British Steel went out of business.

Joanne Lee Cornish

I was born and brought up in the North East of England, at a young age I began to excel in sports, I now live in Malibu California as a well established Personal Trainer and Nutritionist.

Achieving Success
by Connie Garner

What does it take to win a World Title? Is it achievable? Can anyone do it? Or to be successful at anything you are passionate about…

The answers you seek are here, I'm happy to tell you that:

Anyone can do it! And; It is achievable!

But it isn't easy… Nothing worth having is ever achieved easily, nor is it handed to you on a platter.

There are keys to success, neither difficult nor unattainable but a plan you need to stick to and replicate:

- A Plan
- Focus
- Determination
- Hard work
- Sacrifice
- Persistence
- Attitude
- Patience
- Going the extra mile

You have in you the ability to do all of the above and success will follow, in anything you apply that formula to.

I'm going to talk in depth on each of these areas with specific examples of how they led to my success.

My Background

I grew up in Canberra, Australia. I have three brothers all younger than me. My parents separated when I was 7. I played all sorts of sports throughout my school years; Soccer, Netball, Hockey, Basketball, Water

Polo, Athletics.

Looking back now, I used sport as an escape from a difficult childhood; my life was no easy road. I danced outside of school, which was something I loved to do very much. In my junior high years my physical education teacher got me involved in Aerobics classes and I found something I really loved. I was a regular participant, later becoming an Instructor and then a Sport Aerobic Champion.

I then found a love for weight training and in combining Aerobics and Weight training I found the sport of Fitness Competitions and fell in love. I would watch competitions all the time and then competed successfully locally then nationally and later internationally.

A Plan (Your goals and how to achieve them)

You need a plan if you are to achieve anything in an organised and methodical manner – which will lead you to success.

Think of it as getting in your car and knowing where you want to go and deciding to use your navigation system (your plan) or just guessing which way to go. You may get there if you don't use your navigation system or you may get lost along the way. The navigation system (your plan) will keep you on the right track, give you guidance on what you need to do in order to get to the destination (your goal).

You may use vision boards, written plans, sticky notes, project software, whatever you are comfortable with using and what's familiar and easiest for you to follow. You may like a combination of methods.

My plan was in a large A4 folder, which held everything I needed to guide me to success.

The cover page was where I wrote my end goals:
- Complete my University Degree
- Win Australian Fitness Title

- Compete Overseas (I hadn't even dreamed of a World Title at that stage)

These were on the front cover of my folder, I saw them daily. Inside the folder was the roadmap of how to achieve these goals; things like daily training routines, dieting information, special routine moves I was working on, outfit ideas, music ideas, fitness magazines, to do lists and positive inspirational quotes.

Your goals:
- Make sure the goal you are working for is something you really want, not just something that sounds good.
- The important thing to remember here is that your goals must be consistent with your values.
- Write your goal in the positive instead of the negative.
- Work for what you want, not for what you want to leave behind.
- Make sure your goal is high enough.
- Shoot for the moon, if you miss you'll still be in the stars

Focus

Focus is a must to stay on track with your plan and keep moving toward your goals. If you are passionate about what it is you wish to achieve you will find it very easy to focus on what you want.

Determination

The difference between almost and complete success is determination. Many people quit when they are so close to success. On your path to success you will have setbacks, failures, negative influences and self doubt. Your determination needs to be stronger than the negative influences in order for you to succeed. Determination is within you, if it's not apparent then dig deep. When you really truly want something so bad, determination is found.

Hard work

Nobody died from hard work, nor will success come without it...

I had very good role models for hard work growing up, my dad's (I have had a father and a step father since I was 7 years old) both of whom have ridiculously strong work ethics. They are the hardest workers I've ever known, they thrive on keeping busy and achieving outcomes. I had a stay at home mother who did everything in the house.

I have never been afraid of hard work; I've never really viewed anything I do as work. Strange you may think, but when you choose to do things that you love to do and you get paid to do it, not a day goes by where you feel that you work, but rather it's all play.

How much hard work can fitness be? Here's an example of my day (and you wake up and repeat it all again the next day) when training for a competition;

0500 - Wake up, have a strong coffee, pack everything I need for the day and head to the gym

0530 – 0730 - Cardio and Weight training

0800 – 1730 - Work

1230 – 1330 - Run during lunch break

1800 – 1930 - Skills and Flexibility training

2000 - Prepare food for next day

Sleep for 5 - 7 hours.

Training for fitness competitions my payoff wasn't financial; it was achievement that was the pay off. Achievements were getting stronger, more flexible, nailing my routine or getting fitter.

Sacrifice

You just read a typical day and you're wondering, where's time for TV, socialising, partying and other time fillers. Well now you've hit success front on – only through sacrifice do you see results and success. What you sacrifice depends on what you wish to achieve, I never looked at it as a sacrifice. If you have addictions, food, TV, partying etc. then you will see it as a sacrifice and you need to be willing to commit to being able to let go of the old to make way for the new. During this phase of my life I did not have time for TV or partying or eating junk food but I'm absolutely sure that my life is better for that.

Persistence

I can tell you one thing for sure, you can't be successful without persistence. It's about the ability to keep going even when you want to quit. The ability to push yourself where you thought you couldn't go. Persistence is about not accepting failure as an option.

Attitude

Your attitude impacts your success. We all have ways of seeing the world that are influenced by our genetics and our environmental effects, however you can most certainly choose your attitude be it good, bad or indifferent. Let me give you an example, I participated in a competition where it was close first between myself and another girl, in my opinion, she was in front, however this girl was the most unhappy and unfriendly looking person I've come across in all competitions. I am the polar opposite naturally, I was born happy, on top of that I was competing which I absolutely love to do. There were TV crews interviewing us, judges walking around everywhere and not once did I see this girl smile on or off stage. To put it politely she had a bad attitude. It lost her that competition.

Patience

Success does not just happen, it won't come overnight, you will need patience.

Injuries require to be patient, you can't force the healing process, allow it to be time to plan to succeed.

Setbacks come in many forms and often cause frustration, this is when patience is your friend. Ride out whatever setbacks come your way.

There are times when you will think you are ready, prepared, you've done everything you can and you don't win. Hey that's ok, it's happened to everyone! Just be patient and you will succeed

Going the extra mile

Successful people don't do what everyone else does. Sure they may model some traits, behaviours, styles etc. from other successful people but they find a way to go the extra mile, to shake things up, to do things differently. What can you do to go the extra mile towards your own success?

I suggest you surround yourself with positive influences and role models – get a good mentor not someone who tells you what they think you want to hear but someone who will tell it like it is.

Now you have the plan, what will you decide to do with it and the rest of your life?

TRAIN WITH DESIRE, DESIRE TO BE BETTER TOMORROW THAN YOU ARE TODAY.

Love,

Connie Garner

I'm a Miss World Fitness Champion, I'm into fitness. I have two degrees and work in IT and fitness.

Secrets to Having a Mind Over The Matter
by Hilary Hagner

Setting realistic goals and surrounding myself with motivational quotes, scriptures and pictures are what have been my secret tools for success. It was my journey that taught me the long, hard way to set goals and achieve them. My hope is that I am able to help you push past any setbacks and catapult you forward towards your own personal best.

My fitness journey isn't like most others. My fitness journey was birthed out of a desire to earn love and respect for myself. I didn't grow up playing sports; I didn't have an athletic family. In fact, to put it blatantly, I grew up an overweight adolescent. I lost my mother when I was only 8 years old to a sudden brain aneurysm. It left me lost, confused, and very lonely. In junior high school I, like most kids, dealt with a lot of insecurities and anxiety. It wasn't until I started playing basketball and volleyball that I realized how much control I had over my actions. I learned that if I stopped eating then I would lose the weight. I also learned that if I worked out all day then I could expend a massive amount of calories.

In high school, that mindset, transcended to an eating disorder. Bulimia haunted me all the way through my collegiate cheerleading season. It took 5 years for me to finally surrender to extreme fatigue and pure exhaustion which led me to hire a Nutritionist and Personal Trainer. They helped me learn how to be healthy (not skinny). The gym I was training at (at that time) was filled with Bodybuilders and Figure Competitors, so needless to say I instantly became motivated! I thought to myself, "All this time I have been starving myself, I could've been eating and building a beautiful body like these people!?!" I absorbed everything I could from everyone there and got my health under control. That's when

I decided that I wanted to help people find their way to a healthy lifestyle as well, so I became a certified personal trainer. It was in those early days of training that I conceived the dream of one day competing; however, I didn't step on stage until AFTER having two children. My first show was in 2008 and I have been competing ever since. I like to think that my children are what saved me from ever going back to my old roots of insecurities and have given me a whole new sense of confidence and courage.

As a figure competitor or simply someone that wants to take their fitness to the next level, there are challenges you will face regularly. That is why I find it incredibly important to gear yourself up for challenges ahead. One of my favorite quotes is by the legend Arnold Schwarzenegger, "The mind always fails first, not the body. The secret is to make your mind work for you, not against you". In other words, you must keep your mind equipped, empowered, and focused at all times in order to reach your goal. Here are my top five secrets for keeping your mind working for you...

1. Map out your goals on paper. Create in your mind exactly what it is that you desire to accomplish. As long as the physique you are envisioning is your body and not someone else's then your goal is not "too ambitious". No dream is too big or too great! You need to first know what it is that you are hoping to accomplish and then translate that onto paper. Now give yourself a timeline. Will it take five years to reach your goal? Ok, and then write that down. At this time, you now we have a point A and a point B. What will it take in order for you to get there? Write that down too. I found that the more detailed my step-by-step list approach was for reaching my ultimate goal, the more successful I became in the end.

2. Create a Vision Board. I used old magazines to cut out pictures, phrases and quotes that represent exactly what I hope to accomplish in my life. Do not limit your board to just fitness goals though! You will

find on mine a picture of twin babies because as long as I can remember, I have dreamed that one day I would have twins. A few phrases that I have on my board are, "Live Loud", "There are No Limits", and "There's no stopping her". Keep your vision board somewhere that you look often. Mine is hanging in our restroom that way when I am getting ready for my day, I can glance over and pick up a couple phrases to inspire me and awaken my dreams.

3. Self-Talk…out loud! There is something so powerful that happens within yourself when you say out loud everything that you hope to accomplish. I spend a lot of time in my car during the day so while I am on my way to a client's house I declare that, "I am talented, creative, and focused. There is nothing that is going to stop me from conquering my dreams. Doors of opportunity keep opening up for me and doors that lead me nowhere have been shut. I am confident, secure, and victorious. Every day I am one step closer towards my goal."

4. Surround yourself with like-minded friends. There is nothing worse than setting goals and motivating yourself to follow-through with your plan and then get bashed by every person you share your excitement with. Not everyone will rejoice with you. In fact, you will quickly realize that your goals and determination will actually offend a few loved ones. It is nothing personal against you; they are upset because they are not willing to make the commitment like you and in result, they are made at themselves. Being around friends that are aiming towards the same goal as you will actually electrify your dreams and thrust you further along your journey. If you are having a hard time finding people that are like-minded consider looking up inspiring people on Instagram and or www.Bodyspace.bodybuilding.com profiles.

5. Stay current. As you surpass mini goals heading towards your main goal be sure to celebrate your success, but hop back on the road

and keep moving forward. Moving forward may require that you update your vision board. Moving forward may require that you rewrite your self-talk speech. Don't allow yourself to be limited by old mindsets simply because you didn't renew your surroundings. Keep everything current.

You were made for more! You would not be living right now if there wasn't purpose in you. Stand up tall with your head held high. Our obese world needs us to take a stand for health and wellness. Be the one to make a difference for our future. You won't regret it!

Hilary Hagner
I'm a personal trainer. Mother of two and a figure athlete.

You Make Your Own Luck
by Natalie Jill

I remember the day so clearly: It was the middle of the summer on a Sunday and I was walking with my two white labs. I was walking down the street in a neighborhood I loved. At the time, I was 8 months pregnant. Anyone who walked by me that day would have judged and thought I had a perfect life.

I was emotional while I was walking that day and I was crying. At the time, I was working full time as a National Sales Manager for a Medical Device company and I was traveling weekly. It was a Sunday and I was to get on an airplane AGAIN the next morning. The last thing I felt like doing 8 months pregnant was traveling across country at 6AM the next morning.

I was married (unhappily) to someone who had been my best friend. I had gained 50lbs and still had a month of pregnancy to go. I was living in a house I couldn't afford; I didn't know how I was going to pay the bills. I was stressing about maternity leave and how my financial problems would likely get worse.

I was feeling lonely, afraid and out of control and I hated my life. I had always been so excited about having a daughter and now here I was with my greatest wish happening and everything else falling apart all around me. Even worse, my best friend, my husband, was no longer my best friend. My closest girlfriends and my family all lived on the east coast and I was out in California. I felt truly alone.

My Rock Bottom - After my daughter was born matters spiraled out of control. I took a voluntary demotion (so I could stop traveling as much) and my financial problems got worse. The housing market crashed, the stock market crashed, my savings was gone and we filed for divorce.

My dream house couldn't be paid for anymore so I stopped paying the mortgage. My house - something I had invested a lot of my hard earned money in, was going to be gone.

My credit cards were cancelled, my car was having issues, I had to find a daycare so I could work. I had to now share custody of my daughter which meant less time with the one person who meant the world to me. I was overweight, depressed and more alone then I had ever felt and I was 35. Everything I had been years before - confident, fit, successful, happy, was GONE. I didn't know where that girl was. The dream life I had wanted and had was coming to an end.

This is not who I am. I could have given up. All of that could have been solid reasons to be out of shape, unhealthy and even alone today. That was not what I wanted for myself. I wanted to be the person I once was and maybe even better. I did not resort to drugs, alcohol or medications. I did not give up, I did not wallow in my excuses, I did the opposite.

I decided to make my own luck. What was the opportunity in all of this? I could reinvent my life. I listed out my goals. I made a vision board and I decided to practice what I knew would work: to Act as if I was already the person I wanted to become. I DECIDED to do the work. I knew things would work out if I just moved in the direction of success. I would be SUCCESSFUL. I put what I taught in sales for so long into play. I listed out my goals, I put what I knew about fitness and nutrition into play, and I got my body back. I did the work. I did not take short cuts, I DID THE WORK…

Once I had control of my body and my health, things became more clear. I turned my problems into opportunities and made my own luck.

When someone says "it sucks you have to share custody of your daughter" I say "I am fortunate that she has two families that love her and I have an opportunity to have a few nights to myself."

When someone says it "sucks you lost your house" I say "It is AWESOME that I live in an affordable cute house that I can walk to the beach from now."

When someone says it "sucks that you no longer have that high powered job" I say "it is awesome that I spend my days working on my own business and have the freedom to pick my daughter up from school at 3." And when someone says "it sucks that you are divorced" I say "I am so lucky to have found my soulmate at 40."

When you do the work, you work through the process and that in itself is healing. Excuses will not make your life better. Luck does not just happen. You make your own luck.

Natalie Jill
I'm a Fitness, Nutrition and Weight Loss Expert.

Follow Your Heart
by Natasha Jonas

As a child I was never allowed to sit about the house. I was always encouraged to be outside and be active. My fondest memories of my childhood are of playing with my two older male cousins. Being the oldest girl in the house (at that time) I felt I was always in competition with the boys and in order to be accepted and equal I had to be like them. This meant I played a lot of football, climbed a lot of trees, fought and generally enjoyed things considered as 'boys play'. This friendly competition and need to feel equal, I would say was the making of the competitor that you see today.

My love for playing and being involved in sport, led to me watching and following sports, athletes and teams. I don't remember this, but I have been told by my mother that whilst watching an Olympic Games in my pre-teen years, I turned to her and said "Mum, I'm going to be there". This was something I then later repeated to my physical education teacher in secondary school who I would say was another catalyst for me in competitive sports. I have tried so many different sports, and competed at international, county and local levels. There have been many highs and lows throughout my career but I think this will, drive and determination to be a sporting 'somebody' has always subconsciously stayed with me. I never knew how I was going to succeed, all I knew was that I was going to.

There was no better feeling than being able to speak to my mum after my Olympic qualification fight and being able to say "I did it, I'm going to be an Olympian", especially since she remembers me being that child saying I want to be there. The road was long, hard and sometimes the dream felt like an impossibility, but I never gave up, I always believed in myself, gave my all and that kept the dream alive.

Fighting for the biggest plate of food with my cousins or for the control of the tv remote was a daily battle, so you would think naturally that a combat sport would be for me, but it wasn't. Coming from a big family, I always liked to be part of a team and competing as part of a group where there was a joint effort. Boxing was different, there was nobody to hide behind in the Boxing ring, its the ultimate gladiatorial feel of you versus another person, totally different to what I had been use to but adapted too, I had only myself to rely on and I loved it.

I would consider myself to be a strong minded person and have never been easily influenced by others, when none of my friends joined the local boxing club with me, that didn't surprised me and I wasn't scared to go along by myself to a formerly all male amateur club. None of my friends wanted to be boxers, but that didn't bother me, I did. When challenged about my love for sport by friends, family and others I felt that this was right for me and that I'd found my calling and nobody could change my mindset. The more I was challenged the more determined that made me prove myself, I can be a boxer, I will be a boxer and I will be successful and prove you wrong. When it comes to competing sport I have never been your average, it changed me into a different person, this is another me.

The best advice I can give is follow your heart when deciding what it is you truly want from life, don't let nothing or no one deter or influence you from achieving your dreams. It's an old cliché but I do believe that anything is possible. Have a dream, believe you can achieve it, work hard through tough times and you will get your rewards. Do not focus on the how, it does not matter because destiny will always find a way.

Natasha Jonas
I'm a London 2012 Olympian, World bronze medalist, athlete mentor and boxing phenomenon.

Becoming a Better Version of Me
by Christine Keefer

"No matter who you are, no matter what you did, no matter where you've come from, you can always change; become a better version of yourself." – Madonna

Passion, commitment, persistence and self-motivation are the key elements that I have used to achieve my goal of transforming my body and becoming a professional figure competitor. Hello my name is Christine Keefer and I would like to share with you the story of my journey of becoming a better version of myself and how you can do the same.

Like many other young women, I was very insecure about my body image and even suffered from bulimia for a period of time during my adolescence. As a teen, when I saw women with athletic physiques I dreamed to one day look like them. Everyone has dreams; unfortunately not everyone has the courage to go after them. I decided to make my dream to have an athletic physique a reality at the most inopportune time of my life. I was in an unhealthy relationship and my grandmother who was near and dear to me passed away. These two life-changing events propelled me into the world of weightlifting.

At the time I had no idea how much weight lifting would change my life. I was able to find peace, and was able to improve not only my body but my mind and soul. I was able to rebuild what was completely destroyed by the pain from the adversity and insecurities I endured throughout my life. After months of training hard I decided to compete in a figure competition to show off my hard work. I had no idea what I was getting myself into, but it gave me a sense of purpose, which I was lacking.

Stepping on a competitive stage for the first time was very nerve racking. I wish I could tell you that I came out on top at my first show. Fortunately, I did not do well; in fact I didn't even place. This experience set me up for a success that I never thought was possible and I know now that was what needed to happen. If I had won, I would not have appreciated the road that was ahead or the success that followed.

Unlike other times in my life, failure was no longer an option! For the first time in my life I wanted to do better and be better and not settle. In the gym, I found something I could improve on and didn't have to settle for being average. I trained hard to overcome any challenge or obstacle I faced in the gym. For example, I initially could not do lunges with weight. I persevered and never gave up and eventually could do it and was able to add more and more weight over time. Persevering in the gym empowered me from the inside out and it crossed over to other areas in my life. This is something I desperately needed for change to occur and for me to improve and grow mentally, physically and spiritually.

Following my first show, I was determined to prove to myself that I could do better. I set my goals ever higher and picked another show to compete in. I started with setting small goals as simple as being able to do a pull up. By setting small goals I was able to stay focused and motivated between shows. I competed in several competitions that first year and eventually earned a 1st place finish.

Although things were going well for me as a competitor, that was not the case in my personal life. I decided to end my unhealthy relationship that had lasted for ten years. I stepped out on faith and decided to leave everything behind in hopes to find a piece of myself that had been missing. Not only did I have to deal with the painful emotions that were left over from that relationship, I was now a single mother as well. Raising a child alone, dealing with a nasty break up, while continuing to train and compete was challenging. Fortunately, my loving and supportive mother welcomed my daughter Amanda and I into her home and allowed us to live with her for 6 months, until I was strong enough to live on my own. This was a pivotal time in my life and I was able to rejuvenate myself mentally, physically and spiritually and became a better Christian, a better mother and a stronger woman.

Motherhood is one of the greatest joys of my life and I feel that my daughter was God's special gift to me. Being a mother empowered me to become a stronger woman. I was no longer just caring for myself; I now had to care for a child who depended solely on me.

She may not know it yet, but she has given me the strength to survive. Because of her I can now fully appreciate the simple things in life. She has shown me what true unconditional and real love is. It's hard at times for me to understand how God could love someone like me who has made a ton of mistakes and is so far from perfect. Now that I have a child of my own that I love wholeheartedly and unconditionally I can truly understand God's love for me. There is nothing that I wouldn't do for Amanda and nothing she could do to make me ever stop loving her. The parallel between my love for her and God's love for me is amazing. Being a mother also forced me to take a good look at myself in the mirror and has motivated me to strive every day to be the best role model possible for my daughter and other young women.

Trying to balance my role of a single mom, competitor and personal trainer is no easy feat. There are many days where it seems that there are just not enough hours in the day. I am constantly on the go and it feels as though I hardly have time to breathe. With the grace of God and planning ahead I've been able to successfully juggle spending time with my family, training myself and my clients. The success I've had in my roles as a mother, trainer, and competitor has helped me improve my self-confidence and self-esteem significantly.

Prior to assuming these roles I was very insecure and had little to no confidence in myself or my abilities. Learning to love myself despite all my imperfections is a daily battle.

Some days are better than others and much better for me now than they used to be. In order to love yourself you have to be comfortable with who you are. I have had to learn to accept that I am not perfect and that all my imperfections make me who I am. The days when I struggle with this I turn to God for my strength through the Bible, Christian music, or Joyce Meyers broadcast. Within minutes of tuning into one of these sources my spirit is renewed and I am able to continue on with my day.

I hope that by reading this I have helped to inspire you on your journey. No matter what you are going through good or bad, appreciate every moment because all of those moments are molding you to be who God has planned you to be.

I have been fortunate and blessed to be succeeding in life, but all the success in my life is worth nothing unless I can help and inspire others around me. I hope that with God's strength and guidance I can make a difference in the world through others around me. My ultimate goal in life is to encourage, uplift, and inspire others.

Christine Keefer
I'm a caring mother with a true passion for health and fitness and helping others while serving God.

Tough Love on Negativity
by Kimber Kiefer

Jan 2012 was when I decided to take my fitness to the next level and make my dreams my reality. I set my first big fitness goal... bikini competition. What better motivation than knowing you would be walking on stage in a tiny bikini in 5" heels with other gorgeous girls and being judged? It was the motivation I needed to push myself beyond my own limits and out of my comfort zone. I started to learn the true concept of clean eating and the benefits of lifting weights. It was such an amazing journey from beginning to end. It what was started my journey to live a healthy fit lifestyle. I learned so much about myself mentally and physically. It built my self-confidence and made me realize that I have a passion for fitness. It is truly awesome to be able to do something you love and inspire and motivate others along the way! I know competing is not for everyone. It is life consuming and takes some major dedication, motivation, and willpower. You have to find something that motivates you to be better and achieve your impossible. I strongly encourage people to step out of their comfort zone and set goals. The sky is the limit and anyone can do it. Of course, you must believe in yourself and put in the effort and it can and will happen. Everyday in life is a blessing and full of opportunities to make your dreams your reality. Taking chances in life is really about overcoming your fears. Don't let fear hold you back from getting what you want out of life. Making choices and taking chances in life allows you to learn and grow. Know that it is ok to make mistakes and fail; it is actually an important part of being successful.

My lifestyle has completely changed since January 2012. I live a healthy fit lifestyle full time now. I love it and it makes me happy. I must say it has had its challenges though. Life isn't always easy or perfect for anyone and we all have challenges and struggles in our life no matter who we are. We cannot control everything that goes on in our life, but we can control our attitude and how we deal with things. Please know that if you don't surround yourself with positive supportive people it is not possible to be successful. Associating yourself with positive, focused people who lift you higher and that you can learn from will increase your success and happiness in life.

I will be honest, there have been some major changes in my life since I started living my healthy fit lifestyle. I was forced to get a new job and made the decision to remove myself from a negative toxic training environment. It was upsetting and a hard decision to make, but it has helped me learn the importance of finding and focusing on the positive even in the negative situations in life. Remember there are lessons to be learned and growth to be made in every situation. It is what makes us who we are today. "We don't grow when things are easy; we grow when we face challenges."

One of the biggest obstacles I struggled with when my lifestyle changed was dealing with negativity and unsupportive friends, coworkers and family members. You have to remember it is important to keep your priorities in check and balance in your life: family, career, clean eating, training, etc. Not always an easy task. Have you dealt with negative people before? If you have you know how draining it can be. You must help the important people in your life understand how important this lifestyle is to you and how positive it can be. If people are not willing to be positive and support you; reduce contact with some people and you may even have to disconnect completely. Negative people are negative because they lack love, positivity and warmth in their life. You can make the effort to put some positivity and love in their life, but don't waste too much time and energy if they are not accepting. Often, negative behavior is a barrier used to protect them against the world. To approach them, you need to understand where the negativity is coming from: jealousy, misunderstanding or concern.

Jealousy can be very ugly and bring up a lot of negativity. One of the main causes of jealousy is lack of self-confidence. Jealous people put others down to boost their own self-esteem. Some people have a hard time watching others make improvements in their life and get angry and/or jealous. Life is too short and precious to be around people that don't support you and your healthy fit lifestyle. If people are toxic and negative and don't listen to your concerns it is best to eliminate them from your life in any situation. People that love and care for you will want you to succeed in your new healthy fit lifestyle and life in general.

Sometimes others don't understand the process and benefits of clean eating and living a healthy fit lifestyle. We can take the opportunity to educate them and involve them by getting them to work out with you and/or try one of your healthy recipes. If they still do not understand, support you, or respect your feelings, you will have to decide if it is best to decrease contact or completely eliminate them from your life.

Is the negativity stemming from concern? People have a hard time with change in their lives. I have learned through the major changes in my life that change is uncomfortable at first, but it is truly an opportunity to grow and learn. "With every great risk comes great reward." Once others get over the initial shock of the change and see the benefits of your healthy fit lifestyle, they might want to join you. Sometimes you might have to have some patience and give them some time to adjust to the new you. It is important to make an effort with the people that are important to you, but if they don't wish the best for you, it is time to evaluate the importance of them in your life.

Communication is always the best way to deal with an issue. Express your feelings and allow the negative people the opportunity to understand where you are coming from and the importance of this new lifestyle and new you. If they are not willing to accept you for who you are, you don't need them in your life. "Be yourself, because the people that mind don't matter, and the people that matter, don't mind" It is important to make the effort with the people in your life that are kind, love you, and have a positive influence on you and your lifestyle. I always strive to be a positive role model and have positive effects on the lives of others. I am a firm believer in karma, what goes around comes around.

If you want to be successful at living a healthy fit lifestyle, you must surround yourself with people that are positive and supportive. It is not an easy lifestyle and it takes hard work, dedication, and willpower. Many people fail time and time again because they don't create a solid support and accountability system. We all need a system that holds us accountable to our lifestyles, behaviors, habits, and actions and leads us towards our health and fitness goals. There will always be temptations and struggles and sometimes you will give in. Don't get down on yourself if you have a bad day, we are all human. Don't allow yourself to spiral out of control. Always remember tomorrow is a new day to start fresh. Do know that changing your lifestyle often requires changing your environment and the people in it. Having supportive and encouraging people around is a must to be successful. Find a support system that works for you: workout partner (love my workout partner Abi Christine Woodcock), join a fitness group on Facebook, or get a trainer. Having support increases your chances for success. Having someone to support you through your highs and lows is motivating and keeps you both on track. The type of people you surround yourself with has a huge impact on your well being and your mental attitude. A positive mental attitude improves your health, enhances your relationships, increases your chances of success, and adds years to your life. So, surround yourself with people who are positive, who love you, support you, believe in you and do the same for them. You must realize that your mindset and outlook has a huge effect on your level of happiness. "Surround yourself with people who lift you higher and believe in your dreams." My husband and family have been very accepting of the new me and I couldn't do it without their love and support. Always keep life fun and interesting and challenge yourself.

I want to thank Miriam for this awesome opportunity to be part of such an amazing motivating book "Real Talk Real Women". This book is going to be a must have to read over and over for motivation and inspiration. I am a huge fan of strong powerful women empowering each other and that is what Real Talk Real Women is all about. SO honored to be included with all these amazing inspiring ladies.

Kimber Kiefer

I'm a model, fitness guru and bikini competitor. My competition in life is with myself and no one else. I'm always striving to be a better me & push myself beyond my own limits.

The 7 Lessons That Made Me a Champion by Julie Kitchen

My name is Julie Kitchen. I was born on April 19th 1977 in Cornwall, England. Growing up I was extremely shy. As a result, I kept to myself and didn't make a lot of friends and people didn't think much of me.

As I grew older, I went on to win 14 Muay Thai World Championships and became a globally known female martial artist.

These are the 7 lessons that I've learned along the way.

#1. Take Responsibility

A major turning point in my life came when I gave birth to my twins Allaya and Amber in February 1999. When you get children, you put your own life on the back seat and they become your priority. I realised that I now had to take control of my life. I had to learn how to stand up for myself, speak up and take care of them.

The first step is to take responsibility for your life.

#2. Go For Your Dreams

After I had my twins I wanted to lose some baby weight and got addicted to the feeling of training and getting fit. That's when I really became involved in Muay Thai at Touchgloves Gym.

I went on to support one of the junior fighters who had been preparing for a competition with my husband Nathan. When I watched him get in the ring and experienced the lights and the sound and the music I decided that I wanted to have a go at it as well. Not too long after I had my first fight and dominated the fight.

Always go after your dreams.

#3. Never Give Up

My first fight I had no expectations - I just wanted to prove to myself I had it in me. While I won that first fight, out of the first seven I only won 2 and had to endure 5 losses.

Muay Thai didn't come natural to me, it was a lot of hard work. A lot of training. And along the way I've had to overcome a lot.

Never, ever give up.

#4. Learn From Your Experiences

When fighting, for me, it's not about winning or losing. It's about the challenge and the learning experience.

Each fight, whether in the ring or in life, is an opportunity to learn new things. To better yourself.

A loss is not a loss unless you don't learn from the experience. I make it a priority to learn from my experiences.

Try to learn from every experience, whether positive or negative, to continuously better yourself.

#5. Recognise Opportunity

A huge turning point was a visit to London to watch two of the girls who had beaten me before fight each other. It was a really big show for Sky Sports and their fight was the only female fight.

Just before the fight a girl got pulled out because they were fussing over a kilo in weight.

I just had something inside of me that said: "You should fight. You should step in."

I wasn't in fight shape but I gave it my all and beat her every round. That fight really helped my career take off and enabled me to participate in bigger events.

Recognising opportunities and just "going for it" can make a tremendous difference in your life.

#6. Don't Limit Yourself

I was shy and quiet when I was young. People didn't expect much of me. I started fighting very late. Muay Thai didn't come natural to me. People told me I was crazy to get into the ring and fight.

Yet I decided not to limit myself despite all those things.

I'm so happy I listened to my gut and never limited myself. The sport has made me travel and see the world and experience some of the most amazing things.

When I started I never could have imagined that I would be world champion, let alone 14 times world champion. Even now when I write this it seems unreal.

Don't ever limit yourself.

#7. Keep At It

While I've now retired from fighting, my journey is far from over.

Life has many seasons and right now I'm hoping to inspire and play a role in the success of future fighters. I find tremendous pleasure in passing on my knowledge. Aside from my teaching in Holland I travel the world sharing what I've learned through seminars and my involvement in events.

I try to listen to and respond when my fans ask me about certain things. One of the things that keeps coming up is diet so I'm working on a line of sports nutrition products that I stand behind and believe in to help fighters improve their performance.

And who knows what lies in the future!

Keep at it, I certainly will.

Julie Kitchen
I'm known as the Queen of Muay Thai and have won 14 Muay Thai World Championships.

Believe
by Noora Kuusivuori

What an inspiration for me to be a part of this amazing group of women and to be able to contribute to this book. Thinking of what topic to write about for me is easy; I have to share some of my real life story that I feel can show others what believing can do for your life.

My life is absolutely amazing in every area now. Looking back on some situations or parts of my life though, I have overcome things that could break a person. I'll get personal and share a situation that I was in several years ago that I consider a breaking point. At the time I was married and my son was less than a year old. On the surface our lives looked perfect. We were a highly educated couple with successful careers, nice home, tons of travel to nice locations, a healthy baby etc. Reality behind closed doors was not as perfect.

Without making this entire chapter about the negative experiences, I'll summarize how my world came crashing down and how the fairy tale came to an end. I came to find out that my husband had been cheating on me the entire duration of our time together so for 9 years, I had been living a life that wasn't what I thought it was. When I tried to leave him, he would throw me on the wall, strangle me, beat me and lock me in the bathroom so I couldn't leave. He ripped the phones in the house from the wall if I managed to call 911. He slashed my tires so I couldn't drive away. He slashed the tires of the jogging strollers so I couldn't go running with the baby thinking that that way I wouldn't look attractive to other males. He tried to stop me from going to the gym and I wasn't allowed to have any male friends. The last and one of the worst violent episodes happened after I returned home from a business trip with my infant son.

My husband hadn't covered his tracks from bringing prostitutes into our home and I was beaten again trying to leave him. This time I managed to call the police for long enough for them to track the call and my husband was arrested and take to jail. After putting the baby to bed, I sat on the living room floor opening mail from the time that I had been gone. The mail made me aware of another reality that I had not known about. My husband had not only not paid our mortgage and bills from our account for months but also put $100,000 of debt in my name and committed tax fraud worth another $100,000 over several years. All of it came as a complete surprise to me. The following day, I filed for divorce and a restraining order and in response, my husband quit his job and all of that debt, taxes that he owed to the Government, the overdue bills and taking care of our son was on me. As I got home from the Court House, more devastating news followed. I was let go from my position at my job at Johnson & Johnson due to reorganization. There were other horrible things to add that happened but you can picture that my world had crashed already at that point.

That night, I let myself cry and feel all the emotions of disappointment, anger, hurt, betrayal and being scared. For about an hour. Then I looked at my innocent baby boy and knew that I didn't have any time to be down but instead had to make miracles happen. I also knew that the only way that I could do this was if I believed that I could. I focused on believing that everything would not only be ok but that life would be amazing again. I believed that I could get another great job, pay off the debt that was wrongfully made my responsibility, take care of the baby by myself and start over with a clean slate. I believed with every cell in my body, with all my spirit. I let nothing or no one get me down and I grew to be the strongest me that I had been up until that point in life.

Believing made all the difference. I got the amazing leadership position that I believed I would get and although I had to travel a lot, it allowed me the ability to pay off the debt and do it quickly, provide a good life for my son and get over what felt like the end of the world. I did it all with no help as my ex husband hasn't been employed since then and was diagnosed with an illness that makes it unsafe for him to be around a child. I believed that although that life that I thought would last forever was over, I could make life amazing again and that is what I did. That is what I do every single day of life, through the times that have felt difficult and through the days that already feel like a blessing when I open my eyes.

To truly understand the power of my mind and the power of believing has taken me years. I understood that believing was necessary to make my goals and dreams come true but I have since then taken it to another level. I have learned to speed up the process by making my goals very specific with as much detail as possible and then by attaching strong feelings to my goals. I tested this out earlier this year to see if I could make anything happen if I truly put all my faith in it and in myself. I gave myself one day and a very specific goal of bringing in $10,000 that day. I had no idea how I was going to make this happen and no plan before I set the goal in the morning. I visualized bringing in the amount that day and I believed that I could do it and I went about my busy workday as usual. I dropped off my taxes with my accountant that morning and when I checked my email afterwards, I got a message about a modeling job that paid $3,000. The client secured me for that job within an hour. I was still $7,000 short at the end of the workday but I didn't let that stress me out. Instead I re-enforced the feelings of how amazing it would feel to know that I was able to meet my goal. At 6:30pm I got a call from my accountant that I got a tax return of $11,000. The excitement that I felt knowing that I achieved and beat my goal was the same feeling that I felt that morning when I set the goal and decided to just believe that I could do it. I felt and knew that it was not only possible but could be effortless to achieve my goals.

Why did I share these things from my own life? To let you know that if I can do it, you too can do anything if you believe! And when I say anything, I mean anything. Whether you are facing a crisis, big changes, scared about your future or are wanting to do something amazing in life, believe in yourself and in your goals and you will get where you want to be and achieve everything that you want to achieve and more. Think about the people in your life and you'll realize that the people who always seem to be down and have problems also lack faith in themselves and sometimes in everything in life while the successful and happy people that you know are very self confident and believe without a doubt. The only limits in life are the limits that we create for ourselves. Read that sentence again, the only limits in life are the limits that we create for ourselves. Choose to believe and live amazing!

Lots of love,

Noora Kuusivuori
I'm a Silver NYC international fitness model, Muscle Pharm sponsored athlete and a Muscle & Fitness Hers writer.

My Life is a Journey
by Nicole G. Leier

To want something so bad you are willing to go without sleep, to work like you have never worked in your life. To feel the hair on the back of your neck stand up because you are exactly where you are supposed to be. To know this is your birthright.

To not only make the plan but to follow the plan you have laid out for yourself, to continue on until you achieve the one thing you know is rightfully yours. No one is going to carry you over the finish line, no one is going to do the workouts for you, no one but you is going to make sure you do whatever it takes to get the job done. You can ask 1000 people, read 1000 books on health and fitness, however until you are ready and willing to get the job done nothing will happen. I have no answers to the secrets that have got me to this point.

The only thing I can tell you is I am fueled by determination. I want this so bad that it runs through my veins. I want to be the best that only I can be. I have no need to be better than anyone else, only better than what I was yesterday and when I leave this world I want it to be better because I was here. I have a raw desire & will not be stopped.

My life is a journey. I'm constantly learning. It's not about my destination, it's about how I get there. It's about my success and failure along the way. It's about the connections I make, the inspiration I give and receive. The goals I set guide me along this path, they give me structure and focus, they keep me grounded. But there is no 'end' goal, on this journey. Each milestone achieved is a new beginning, a new opportunity. What have I learned? Where have I come from, and where do I feel the desire to go next? I'm constantly re-plotting my course, and always, always experimenting. I'm learning that it's not about the goals I set, it's the growth that happens along the way. Sometimes it's even about how I don't accomplish what I set out to. Instead, it's about all of the little things along the way.

I'm learning that I can only see so far ahead at any given time. So I set my course, I give it my all, and I spend my time enjoying the ride.

Every tiny step adds up to so much more. And that's the journey.

Love & light,

Nicole G. Leier
I'm an internationally renowned actress / writer / personal trainer / creator.

Taking a Chance
by Fatima Leite Kusch

It was 2004 when I took the biggest risk of my life and created the career of my dreams from scratch. I had been working for a while at a job that I thought was going to be my ideal career. Unfortunately, this path was nothing like I had anticipated. After the first year, I was showing signs of becoming the person I knew didn't want to become. I was suddenly a negative person and it showed up in all areas of my life. I came home every evening feeling a weight of anxiety and stress. On one of these nights when I had come home full of my usual work-related complaints, my husband asked me, "Why do you keep going back if you're so unhappy? You spend most of your life there – it's not worth the stress."

That comment made me stop and consider where I was going and who I was becoming. I thought, "I spend five days a week here, usually at least eight hours per day. What am I getting from this? What does it do for me?" Sadly I wasn't getting anything from this – this was actually making me toxic and I was bringing it home and letting it damage my personal life. Something had to change whether I was ready for it, or not.

I was hardly ready and the scariest part was deciding how I was going to make the shift. Yes I was in a position where I could do anything I wanted, but it was on me to make it work and make an income. How could I come up with a new dream career path when this toxic job was supposed to be what I wanted? I could have simply changed employers and remained in the same industry, but that would have inevitably bred the same negative and unhappy girl I didn't want to be anymore. I exhausted all options and the only career change I could imagine involved health and fitness. At the time I was training for my second fitness competition. This was my only other passion, plus I had already gained credentials in sports nutrition and personal training. This felt like a good fit and a good decision but with this also meant I would lose my benefits, and consistent salary as well as a stable job. Once I left, there would be no turning back. This was scary!

I knew that I wanted to be my own boss. I also knew it isn't easy starting new as a trainer without any clients. But I was willing to try. I was confident that my strong work ethic and willingness to do whatever it takes would carry me through succeeding my own business. The more I considered it, the more comfortable I was with the idea of helping others with their fitness. After much thought and discussion with my husband, I finalized that decision and took the plunge.

The plan was to give myself a few months to see what it was like being my own boss. If it did not feel right, I would then fall back on a position in a gym setting or something similar. Words can't describe how determined I was to not have to go that route.

So, I left my job and became a self-employed trainer. How was I going to get clients? I was terrified of failure – terrified of making a bad decision. It certainly wasn't the safe choice for a stable career. On top of that, my husband was preparing to take care of our monthly expenses fully until my business progressed. How long was that going to take? There were so many unknowns. I don't like the feeling of having to rely on others, which made the change even more uncomfortable.

It was in this first week of self-employment that I went for a walk with an old colleague. She happened to ask for some help losing weight.

Coincidentally, one of my first ideas was to start a boot camp class. I offered to sign her up for an extremely cheap price in hopes of drawing in more potential long-term clients and to gain experience working with various people. She shared the opportunity with a few friends and sooner than later I had too much interest to hold just one class. I wanted to ensure they were all getting the most value out of their class, so I set up 2 classes of 10 girls each. From there we would schedule 1 month of training at a time. Each time I started a new month I increased the price. I LOVED helping people. It was so much fun! It was often challenging but so rewarding.

By Fall of that first year, the outdoor classes were ending. I picked up some new personal training clients from those contacts I had made through Spring/Summer classes. Then the business just kept expanding from there. Each business decision I made was always based on the needs of my clients. That seemed to work well and still works for me to this day.

I've gone from teaching fitness classes to mentoring women and coaching them through modeling, industry branding, competition prep and lifestyle transformations. It's been 7 years since I turned my life right-side up. There has never been a time when I regretted taking this chance. The journey has been challenging but also very rewarding. I truly love what I do now and cannot imagine what kind of person I would be today if I had not left that toxic job. I feel blessed to be coaching women from all over the world and seeing them through achievements they never dreamed were possible.

Taking a chance has brought me a business that I am proud of, amazing people that I am surrounded by, daily rewards in my work life, and most important overall happiness in my day to day living.

Fatima Leite Kusch
I'm a Canadian celebrity fitness model, WBFF Pro Diva Fitness Model, Strong Fitness Magazine columnist, owner of Blessed Bodies Fitness & founder of Blessed Little Sisters (non profit teen athlete scholarship program.)

Finding Your Passion
by Amy Mac

Growing up, I wanted to be a number of things: an astronaut, a CEO, a Broadway musical star and a lawyer. My life has taken lots of twists and turns and many people along the way have rolled their eyes at the fact that I've changed career directions many times and have jumped from city to city across the U.S. For those people that thought I was scattered or hap-hazard, I hope they are starting to realize that it was all calculated chaos. With a great deal of hard work and an amazing support system, my journey is starting to make sense.

Let's roll back and talk about the frustration of knowing that you are capable of doing amazing things but have no idea what they will be and how to set that in motion. I grew up with my parents encouraging me that I could be anything I wanted to be, and they still do. I went off to college as Pre-Law and then changed to Business before I even moved into the dorm. I didn't blend well with the uptight business students - let's say I'm a little too energetic for their liking. So that landed me in the career counselor's office taking every personality trait test in existence that would tell me where I belong. Turns out that I'm exactly in the middle. This sounds like a good thing but according to the lady, it is the worst place to be because I'm perfectly balanced between creative (love of dance and music) and structured (my love of organization, event planning and running businesses). She then explained to me that no matter what job I would hold, I would always be a bit unhappy because there was no job in the world that allowed someone structure and creativity. I wish I could go back and punch that woman, seriously. Who says that to a concerned and confused 20 year old? So I left in tears and called my parents to wallow. My dad very simply said, "Well, if you love fitness and dance and you love to plan and organize things, why don't you just run a fitness/dance studio? That would be the perfect balance of all the things you like." Leave it to the people that know you best to really tell you what you should do with your life. So that led me to the major of Organizational Leadership and Supervision with a minor (unrecognized) in Dance. I was off to a good start.

Let's sum up the years spent as a banker, starting our first company (t-shirt printing), hip hop dancing in Chicago and fitness training in Nashville and San Francisco by saying that I learned skills in all of these ventures and each one led me closer to what I did and did not want to spend the majority of my time doing. Once in San Francisco, I was doing fitness training both in the club, privately and corporate programs. I loved and still love fitness and personal training. Being able to educate and help people change their lives for the better has just always been the most rewarding and awesome experience. When my husband started Podcast Alley, I started a fun little audio podcast called Fitness Attack with Amy Mac. This was a daily 60-second health and fitness tip show. It quickly became popular in iTunes and that show went on for over 500 episodes, with millions and millions of listens. A side effect of that show was that I began doing voiceover work and still do it to this day! (To all the people that said I couldn't make a living by talking - Ha!)

Podcasting got bigger and video podcasting became the new thing. I started my video show, Fit Life, which is still in production and has been syndicated and distributed through more channels than I can recall. I remember checking the stats daily to see how many views an episode had and it was so exciting to have a new subscriber. Those days were many years ago and while I still appreciate every viewer and comment, it is overwhelming to think of how many that has been over the last few years. Yikes! Taking a minute to reflect on that is very surreal, so thank you for indulging me.

If you've stuck around this long (thank you!), you are probably wondering why we are recounting the last 15 years of my life and the point of the story in general. I completely understand so I will try to move it along as quickly as I can. My chapter is capped at 1500 words, so rest assured knowing you are ½ way through!

During our 5 years in San Francisco, I was challenged beyond belief by the people surrounding me. I was a personal trainer when I started the podcasting thing. I began doing more on camera and voiceover work and then started working on a higher level in the production world. I started with content acquisition for a media company and then moved up to running the women's network. This meant I got to use all my creative skills starting shows, making channel lineups and lots of script writing.

I also got to use my organization skills for arranging auditions, studio scheduling and every other production detail that was needed. Producing people, places and props is hard work! In addition to those tasks, I was still able to do fitness projects, "perform" on camera and publish 2 fitness tip books. It was the most frustrating, exhausting and rewarding years of my life. I really began growing up and becoming the person I wanted to be. There is not a day that goes by that I don't use something that I learned from those years.

My mission since the early 2000's has been to give people the knowledge to make healthier choices throughout their day, to maximize their workout and give them that information in a concise, entertaining format. That has always been the driving force for all of my fitness content and it has been amazing to be a part of people making their lives better. Now while that all still remains true, I have moved into the next phase of my journey.

I now own a video production company in Nashville, TN, where I live with my husband and son (as I write this, he is just 5 months old!). It turns out that while I was creating all of those fitness videos, people started to appreciate the entertaining style in which we delivered information. We started being approached by other companies wanting us to create great marketing, sales, product launch or tutorial videos for them with that same energy and style. It started out as side gigs that helped us pay the bills and purchase new equipment and then one day my partner and I looked around and realized that we had become a video production company! We embraced it because we had always loved the production side and could still do our regular content creation. Now if you've paid attention, then you've noticed that it all seems to be coming together, almost like it was planned.

I run my own company so while I don't call myself a CEO, I don't have to answer to anyone else. I get to organize lots of things everyday by producing videos and managing clients. The banking background has definitely helped with some of the basic operations of running and growing a business and I get to jump up on stage on occasion for my own videos, as well as on-camera talent for other projects. Not to mention the creativity that is needed to be able to envision the final project before it is even scripted.

Well, I think we've finally gotten to the point of the story - I hope you find it worthwhile!

I have never known what I wanted to be when I grow up and I still don't. I never fit into the mold that most people thought I should fit into and I think I've done just fine without it. I could go into clichés about taking the road less traveled or making lemonade out of lemons but that would be lame. The real point is: Be true to yourself. Do what you love. I have lived through the rolled eyes at Christmas parties and the jokes about my various business cards and that you could never write my address down in pen. I have spent more time crying in the shower about what I'm supposed to be and where I should do it than I will ever care to calculate. The point is, that I seized every worthy opportunity that was presented to me and I took something, even if it was just the memories, away from it and I'm better for it. My experiences and my random assortment of skills are what make me: ME. As I sit here writing this, I'm looking at a poster on the wall that says, "If you work really hard and are kind, amazing things will happen.

I think that is the perfect line to finish this chapter.

Amy Mac
I'm a personal trainer, fitness personality, author and video producer.

Dreaming Big
by Bridget McManus

As a child I was enamored with "The Carol Burnett Show". At three years old, I would watch reruns of the legendary variety show as I lay on my parent's living room rug. I stared, mouth agape, inches away from our small color TV and ogled at Burnett and her circus of cast members. I, like millions of other dreamers, wanted to be Carol Burnett.

When you're a kid you don't usually think of the logical steps to reach success, you just want something. I wanted to be Carol. I wanted to stand center stage in front of a crowd. I wanted to make people double over from laughter. I wanted to wear all those Bob Mackie costumes.

Thirty years later, I have traveled the world performing as a professional comedian. I also have more costumes than any sane person should. My collection ranges from caveman to Bride of Frankenstein. I feel very fortunate to be able to live my dream every day and I truly believe everyone has the capability to do the same.

The key to following your dream is to allow the river of life take you where you're supposed to end up. So many times we try to control the outcome of events and we think we've failed at something just because the end result doesn't arrive in the package we're expecting. We might not win an Academy Award by the age of 30 or be the first person to land on Mars, but it doesn't mean we should turn our backs on our true callings.

Things weren't always easy for me. I've struggled with weight most of my life fluctuating between 130 to 200 pounds. I was never cast in a high school play, and growing up I was bullied for being different. As I waded through the waters of life, I attended three different universities, starting with a major in kinesiology and eventually obtaining a bachelor's in drama at New York University's Tisch School of the Arts.

After graduating high school I thought I should get a practical degree, one that would make money, instead of becoming a struggling actor. I attended a small teaching school in New Hampshire focusing on kinesiology (the scientific study of human movement), with the goal of helping children who were struggling to lose weight. Even though I did well in school, I knew that studying science was not what I was supposed to be doing. I told the head of the kinesiology department that I wanted to transfer to another school so I could be a performer. I wanted to be a comedian. The woman shook her head and told me that I was being unreasonable. She said I needed to finish my degree because it was impractical to be an artist, and besides I wasn't funny anyway. Even though I knew she meant well, I found her words to be hurtful. So I heeded her warning and stayed in school. One night as I lay in bed, I asked for a clear message to be delivered to me as I slept. I was riddled with self-doubt and needed a sign from the ethers. When I woke up the next morning I had a clear vision of leaving school.

I moved back in with my parents and for a few months I attended a local college as I tried to find my footing. One day, just in passing at a coffee shop, I overheard a young woman bragging about getting into New York University's prestigious Tisch School of the Arts. I remember her high-pitched voice declaring, "If you want to be a star you need to go to New York." I had never heard of this school before but I thought, hey, if this girl can do it so can I! Months later, I arrived in New York for my audition into this magical school that I was convinced would fix my life. I nervously paced the hallway lined with young thespians, all dressed in black. In stark contrast, I was barefoot in a white tee shirt and khakis. Once again I was different. But to my surprise and delight, the admissions officer was looking for someone who was different. I was one of the 16 people in the world (out of the thousands who auditioned) to be accepted into NYU's Spring transfer program. I felt special, like I belonged. I loved my new college life, but soon fear set in. What happens when I graduate? What if I can't make a living being an artist? I was tiptoeing into the shallow pool of my dreams, so in my last year of school I changed my specialty from acting to directing, thinking that it was more practical route to take.

After graduation, doors didn't open up for me as I hoped. My drama degree was pretty as it hung framed on my wall, but it didn't provide any automatic opportunities. I struggled as a waitress, interned at an off-off-off Broadway theater and I moved around, a lot. I left New York for New Jersey then Connecticut then finally ended up moving across the country to the west coast. At the age of 23 I fearlessly (and recklessly) moved to Los Angeles, California. With no savings and no job prospects, I crashed on my friend's living room floor for three months as I tried to hunt down work, any work. It was a very difficult time. I accrued a lot of financial debt and the massive pool of talent that resided in Los Angeles drowned what was left of my former "big fish in a little pond" ego. I eventually got a job as an assistant on a TV show, then starting making commercials, then movies, all on the production side, using my head rather than following my heart. I was bobbing up and down through the pool of life; at night working as an improv actor and stand up comedian and then returning to my office job exhausted every morning.

At the age of 28 everything changed unexpectedly. I was newly single after a long relationship. I left everything from my old life behind, my beloved pet and all of my belongings, and started anew in a studio apartment in Hollywood. I bought a used bed online, which doubled as my couch since there was no place to put furniture in the micro-box where I now lived. I worked seven days a week for a difficult boss and then spent my nights out at comedy clubs trying to make a name for myself. Slowly but steadily, I was picking up steam. I was interviewed for a website article entitled "Female Comedians You Don't Know But Should." From that little mention, I was scouted to be a guest on a weekly video blog. As that internet show became more popular, I was asked to create my own online show. From within my tiny apartment I birthed "Brunch with Bridget," a weekly talk show in which I interviewed female celebrities from my bed in my studio apartment. Each episode was a simulated slumber party, complete with pillow fight. The show became a hit and went on to garner a Logo Network New Now Next Award for Best Vlog Ever. Soon after, I started to get big named guests to interview and my rinky-dink show shot out of my sad little studio apartment was then broadcast on the Logo television network on Friday nights. In less than a year from its inception, I was now producing, directing, editing and starring in my own talk show. Strangely enough, it was hitting rock bottom that propelled me to create my own television show.

"Brunch with Bridget" was just the beginning of my life as a full-fledged performer. Since then I've been able to work on network TV shows (sometimes wearing a leotard and legwarmers), starred in three comedy specials, headlined at resorts all over the world and I continue to fulfill my goal of being a performer. I'm not rich, I'm not famous but I'm living my dream, costumes and all.

As I look back at my humble beginning as a chubby child rolling around on my parent's living room rug, nothing has turned out as I expected. Nothing at all, but that doesn't matter because I couldn't imagine anything as good as how my life is actually unfolding. Who knows what will come next? Carol Burnett famously said, "When you have a dream, you've got to grab it and never let go." So I encourage you (yes, you, the person reading this) to dream big, but more than that I challenge you to dream bigger than you have ever before.

Miriam Khalladi

Because, hey, why not?

Bridget McManus
I'm a professional comedian and actress.

Creating the Life You Love
by Lindy Olsen

For the first time in my life I am happy with myself, I am finally comfortable in my own skin and I love life. This is a statement that I am proud to be able to say, and if you'd asked me nine years ago how I felt about myself, my answer would have been very different indeed. To tell the truth, my story starts the same as a million others, but the choices I made and the small changes I adopted changed my entire world… I'm no different to any other person, I'm not special or lucky, I just had a dream that I didn't let go of.

Transforming yourself and your life…dreams CAN come true!

No matter how long it's been since you've dreamed it…

No matter how "unrealistic" it seems…

Your impossible dream may just be POSSIBLE after all!

Fear of failure…

For as long as I can remember I have had an issue with my weight. It began in high school, when my focus shifted from sport to study. I became the girl at school who was literally the "butt" of everyone's jokes! I was told regularly that my rear end had its own "postcode". I used to laugh it off at the time, ever careful to hide my feelings. To others it was just a bit of "harmless" fun, but it bit deep into my self worth and as I grew older I found myself making fun of my rear, just so I got in before anyone else did.

Up until April of 2003, I was relatively lazy and a comfortable size 14. I was not motivated at all to keep fit. I now know this was mainly due to a combination of studying late at night, little activity and lots of bad food choices. It wasn't long before these habits began to have a detrimental effect on my body and before I had even realised what was happening to me I had ballooned out to 89kg (196.2 pounds).

Feeling insecure about myself and my body had become a way of life. I just accepted it and for a long time used every excuse I could think of to convince myself it wasn't my fault. I think I tried just about every weight-loss pill and diet miracle I could get my hands on - but kept getting bigger and bigger. I needed to find help…fast. I made the decision to get some professional help, found a personal trainer, saved my money and started training two weeks later.

It wasn't long before I started thinking it was all too hard and I didn't have the time, energy or money to continue. Failure was staring me in the face once again, and I remember sitting on the edge of my bed, tears welling in my eyes. I started thinking about all the things that I hated about myself and why I always seemed to get nowhere fast. There were so many reasons I could think of why it just wouldn't work, and my lack of results seemed to be at the top. Later, it would become very clear that I always stopped before I really got started. I was extremely impatient and never did anything long enough to see any significant changes.

Many of the people I meet and have connected with over the past 10 years have similar stories. Many of them often question themselves as to why they find it so hard when everyone around them seems to be doing it all so easily. Guess what, they're NOT! Most successful "transformation" stories are from people who have made exercise part of their lifestyle on a daily basis and these same people live and breathe the benefits. Many others start out with the greatest intentions but somehow, somewhere along the way, lose momentum. There is always an unavoidable crisis or an excuse that suits.

The truth is that until you can identify the real issues that are holding you back, you may be fighting an uphill battle. Acknowledging your weaknesses can be very confronting but if you stick at it, the good news is that you can start to make some real progress.

Six must-dos before making any changes in your life...

ASK - Ask yourself what you really need in order to succeed. Ask yourself what could stand in the way of your progress so that you have a plan to combat it. Our best advice often comes from our most powerful connection to ourselves, our intuition. Listen to your body.

PREPARE - Be prepared for change. Know how you will tackle the hurdles or obstacles that arise. Know what you want and what results you expect to achieve. Know what you are prepared to do for yourself, before giving your time, energy, and commitment. Be focused on your goal and make a promise to yourself that you will allow yourself the time you need to succeed.

BE READY - Being emotionally and mentally ready are vastly different things from being prepared. If you are not ready to accept a few small changes, your plan may take on a direction of its own. Both your mind and body need to be prepared for the changes you are about to make.

TIME - If you really want to make any changes in life you cannot sit and wait for it to be handed to you on a silver platter (although that would be nice). You have to take control of your future success and create your own destiny. Make yourself the biggest promise you've ever made: a promise to BELIEVE in yourself, TO NEVER GIVE UP on your dreams, your goals or your desires! Plan a way to get there and give yourself a realistic timeframe and reach for the stars! Nothing is impossible with a little patience and time if you only try!

FOCUS - No matter what happens in your life, never lose sight of your goal. If you really want to feel better, you must believe you can, if you need help... ASK! Find people who inspire and motivate you to help you keep going… especially when the going gets tough.

SUPPORT - Find someone who really understands you and what you want to achieve. It's not ideal at all jumping from coach to coach, or to not stick to a training / fitness plan long enough to decide if it works for you! There is NEVER a one-size-fits-all plan, so don't expect a pre-designed, cookie-cutter style program to get you the results you really deserve! If your coach is unable or unwilling to answer ALL your questions… GET A NEW COACH!

Above all, GET STARTED NOW!

So… how do you take the next step?

So you're ready to go, you know where you're going and how you're going to get there. So why can't you follow it through? Unless you actually become "conscious" of your goal, you may still find the whole thing very daunting. The day I started becoming conscious of the habits that seemed to be hindering my progress was the day I took control of the wheel. Long before I could actually see things starting to change, I felt more energetic and my clothes were becoming more comfortable. Above all, I actually started feeling good about myself and my life. I have to confess, if I had any idea that wanting to lose a little bit of weight would eventually lead me to compete in front of 400 people wearing a g-string, win several bodyshaping titles and feel this fantastic, I probably would have told you that you were dreaming!

What a lot of people don't understand is that absolutely anyone can compete or stay in great shape all year round! However, only a few ever continue past their first year or maintain a physique that they are truly happy with year-round. Competing requires incredible drive, determination and above all total commitment. The end result you see on stage usually takes months of preparation and even years of weight training to achieve and is far from everyday reality. Competitors rarely maintain their "stage" figures and some only compete once or twice a year. There is always a constant pursuit for perfection and unless you realise that life is rarely perfect, you may end up feeling somewhat disappointed. It is not perfection that we should be seeking but merely peace within ourselves.

Living and loving life…

How life has changed in only nine short years - I no longer hate the physique on the person I see staring back at me in the mirror, I am not in competition shape all year round, however I really try to encourage others to love who they are and live and love life the way they deserve!

Yes, I still love my cheese cake and chocolate just as much as anyone else, but I am living proof that if you make a few small adjustments here and there, you can literally have your cake and eat it too!

So many people of all shapes and sizes just need a helping hand to realise they can achieve anything they desire, if they only try. People who overcome adversity and hardship continue to inspire me with their heartfelt stories of personal success. I am both blessed and privileged to share some small part in their journey.

Make yourself one promise… Don't wait for that perfect time to start… or for the next perfect day. Kick off your next challenge now and take that "long-lost" dream off hold… take the first step, make a start, as that's all it takes to change your life.

Creating a life you love…

The road not travelled is full of regret, but the road you know can only take you where you've already been. Making an improvement in your life is as simple as making a choice. This choice is making a conscious decision to reach your goal by working towards it. For those of you who are willing to make a small contribution to yourself, each and every day, you will succeed.

The hardest thing you will have to endure is not the challenges of your life, nor the colour of your skin. It's not your age or even that person close to you who's convinced that your dreams and aspirations are a waste of time. Without doubt, these challenges will need your attention, but by far the biggest challenge you could ever face is your own self-doubt, lack of commitment, and fear. Getting started is the single most positive step you will ever take.

So here is my message… Believe in Yourself, Get moving and Get Gorgeous from the inside out!

Lindy Olsen

I'm a 5 x times natural world champion in figure sculpting, fitness ambassador and lifestyle and fitness coach.

Rewriting the Story of Your Life
by Marzia Prince

When people meet me today, they assume that I had the best upbringing because of my current situation. I am not going to lie, I am very blessed right now and I love my life today. I hear "Wow, you are so lucky!" WHAT?! Lucky? What are they talking about? I worked my tail off to get to this place in life. Let's get real here, life is not a Disney movie with a fairy tale ending that we were groomed to believe growing up. Life throws us challenges that we have to grow through every day. Sometimes it is easy and we are on top of the world and sometimes it completely sucks. It is what you do right now to handle your current situation that will determine if you succeed, stay in limbo, or fail.

My current situation has nothing to do with luck. The reality is that I grew up in a very strict military catholic family. My dad was an immigrant from Mexico who joined the Air Force at 18 in hopes to live a better life in America and my mom was one of six children born to Nebraska farmer. They were so young when they got married and had me, they were 21 years old. My mom had the 4 of us within 8 years. My parents raised us like little soldiers. There was very little love or positive affirmation in my household. We never heard "good job" or "love you honey". To be quite honest, my parents were miserable. They were struggling with their marriage, finances, and raising a family. My three siblings and I felt the negative pressure growing up, especially in high school. We walked on pins and needles trying not to make our parents mad at us.

I heard 2 things growing up quite often in my household. 1) No, you can't do that and 2) No, we can't afford that. Years of hearing no over and over being played my head make me think "When I am old enough to move out, I vow to live the opposite of my parents!" I did not want their unhappy stressful life. My childhood was not a happy memory for me. Don't get me wrong, I have had some positive memories, but the negative ones outweigh the positive ones. Yeah, I used to wish that I had I had the perfect family. In fact, I used to lie to people and tell them I had the best family and put on a fake smile to the world. I was embarrassed to tell people my parent about my unhappy childhood. I knew it was only a matter of time before the truth makes its way out. I mean, I couldn't lie forever, could I?

Besides feeling the stress of my parent's daily struggles, we had the worst nutrition. Between my dad being Hispanic and my mother being a Nebraska farm girl, we had a combination of traditional Mexican food and hearty home cooked meals with lots of butter and gravy. Also, during high school, I worked at McDonald for three years. I ate that junk almost every day. So, between being unhappy, I had horrible nutrition. I was not the picture of health back then.

I had issues. Here I was a young girl with a ton of childhood issues from my upbringing trying to make it in the world. I was very angry for years. I dated the wrong men, I hung out with the wrong friends, and I thought this was the card I was dealt in life. I had no education on eating the right foods; therefore I was eating processed foods on a daily basis. I had negative self-talk. How else was I supposed to talk to myself? I didn't know how to believe in myself. I never heard positive self-talk at the time, I don't think I would have believed myself at the time if I did say something positive. In fact, when I looked around my life at that time, I was miserable. I was a product of my parents and my environment. I told myself I would change years ago but never put it to action. I complained too long for too many years.

Then one day I decided the pity party was over. I wanted to change my life. I was about 24 when I made the biggest decision in my life. I wanted a new life. I wanted to be happy. I wasn't happy with my current situation and I knew I needed to change it. So I moved to a new city, got a new job, made new friends, started reading books to educate myself, and went back to school all on my own with no help. I read a lot of self-help books and started working out. Day by day I felt like I was rehabbing myself to be the best me I could be. As time went on, between going to college and educating myself (reading a ton of health and fitness books), I was feeling better overall. I knew I was on the right path to living a happier life.

The point of my story is not to make you feel sorry for me or to throw my parents under the bus. That was how my parents knew how to deal with their life at the time. It was one of the hardest times of their lives. They didn't know the consequences of their actions and words would affect their children into adulthood in a negative way. My story is to show you that you have it within you to change your current situation if you really want to. For me, I was tired of living a miserable life every day, it got me nowhere. There was something in me that said "Marzia, you can be happier than this." And that is what I did. If you have it within you to change your current situation whether it be your love, life, career, your health, or your social circle, you can do it. It takes time. My goal back when I was miserable was just to be happy. After changing certain factors in my life, I was on my way to happiness. Only I could change myself. I couldn't blame anyone but me.

Today at 39, I feel blessed. My life now is everything I dreamed about when I was 24 and much more. I would never have believed the negative little girl who worked at McDonald would ever be Ms. Bikini Universe or a fitness model today. Life is what I made it. Happy. It took me years to get here but it was so worth all the life lessons and failures. I rewrote the story of my life day by day and still continue to do so now.

Dig deep inside yourself to make the changes you need for your life.

Your life depends on it. Happiness is part of being healthy. You are a product of the choices you make right now. Go out there and find your happiness.

Marzia Prince
I'm an international fitness model and the creator of Healthy Housewives.

Achieving Success as a Figure Competitor by Louise Rogers

My journey into fitness started when I was a teenager. I always had an ability to train hard and achieve a degree of success in sport whilst in school. In those days my dreams were more focused on competing in an Olympic sport, like sprinting or hurdles. My dreams of going further in this direction were scarpered when I became unwell. For a long while I couldn't exercise properly and I became rather disinterested. When I reached 18 I started attending a gym with my sister. Ironically my sister was training to be a fitness instructor but she was too young to enter the gym on her own so I had to accompany her. Without too much effort I quickly lost some weight and started enjoying exercising again.

After finding enjoyment from attending the gym with my sister I decided to study to become a personal trainer. I figured it would be a great way to earn some extra money whilst at University and I figured it would be fun because I enjoyed training. Soon after I qualified I went to work for a local gym – this was back in 2003. Whilst in the gym I was partnered up with a gentleman training for powerlifting. He introduced me to 'proper' weight training and at last I felt that I had found something I could possibly pursue further, although in which direction I wasn't certain.

One day we were sat at the desk in the gym and my colleague was reading the 'Muscle and Fitness' magazine. Despite my enjoyment of training I hadn't bought the magazine before. He was reading about the Miss Olympia competition which I hadn't heard of. He began to show me pictures of a new class which had been introduced called Professional Figure. To this day I remember seeing Monica Brant and Davana Medina and thinking – this is what I want to do, "I'm going to be a professional figure competitor". Although I could not comprehend how they looked so incredibly fit and how this was possible. I immersed myself in the sport – including the diet, training, learning about the class, learning my route to compete and become a pro. It was certainly a learning curve and I tried various training methods, wacky diets all in a hope to improve myself.

Years past, all the while training and dieting hard. During this time I planned to do a local bodyfitness competition. This would be my first step into competition. During my first attempt to diet down for a competition I caught the flu and I remember feeling rather disheartened. However I rescheduled it and began working towards another competition. Again, with most aspects of my life if I am committed to something I will absorb myself in it totally. I trained ridiculously hard and whilst nervous I just hoped I could give a good account for myself.

It came to my first competition – 5 years after I had first discovered Pro Figure… I competed and won the bodyfitness qualifier which meant I qualified for the British National Championships. I suppose my preparation for it took over my life to some extent, although appreciate I was studying another degree at this point and also working full time. I prioritised my life and everything worked around my training. During this time I kept my physique under wraps and privately tracked my progress with my coach and my partner. Everything remained a secret until the British Championships. I prepared everything meticulously, although I had not expected to win by such a large point score. I clearly remember winning the British Championships in slow motion. To some extent I had made one dream come true, but my goal was to turn professional.

After this point I was given a few opportunities to compete internationally and due to my University exams I opted to compete at the World Championships. This is arguably the most difficult amateur competition in women's fitness/figure/bodybuilding. You're competing with the best amateur athletes in the world and I made it my mission to try and give it everything I had to win a pro card. I know I was up against incredibly talented women and I was aware that so far no woman had managed to win a pro card at this level from the UK. In some ways I didn't expect anything, but at the same time I could not accept failure. Reaching this point had taken me 6 years, 6 years of consistent training and commitment to a goal.

The World Championships took place in Italy in 2009… I went there proudly representing the UK with a small, but great team! The competition was held over several days and we went through a number of rounds to reach the finals. My surprise came when I was on the coach back at the hotel with the other competitors and they mentioned that when we get back to the hotel we will find out who is in the finals. At this point I realised I would know whether I had turned professional. It was the most nerve racking moment when I walked into the hotel and realised our names were pinned to a board indicating if we had reached the finals. Even now I can be tearful when I recall the moment; I could not check my name because I was fraught with nerves. My partner went up to the board and came back to me with tears streaming down his face, he said "you have done it my girl – you're a pro". The words stunned me and for a few moments I sat down quietly, a little tearful but feeling very proud of myself. It took time to realise what I'd achieved and that I had accomplished a goal I'd been working towards for so many years.

After this I realised that I would be starting a whole new journey into the professional figure scene. From this point I would eventually like to compete on the Olympia stage… whether that will happen I don't know. But I have enjoyed the journey so far.

My dream eventually became my reality, although it's not happened with luck. I have worked hard, remained determined and I committed myself to a goal. I truly believe that if you work hard enough and don't give up you can achieve success in everything you wish if you just want it enough.

Louise Rogers
I'm an IFBB professional figure competitor from the United Kingdom.

Putting the Love in Glove
by Hedda Royce

My name is Hedda Royce. I have been asked to write my story. Since I don't consider myself a writer, let me begin with an apology for any dangling participle, or worse that may be contained herein. With that expressed I submit the following and hope that you find the read both interesting and enjoyable. This is my "so far but much more to come" journey.

I consider myself to possess an ample amount of self-esteem and confidence. This is probably because my parents were nurturing people who showered lots of love on both me and my sibling, an older brother. I guess you could say that I idolized my brother. He was good at everything and I wanted to be just like him. If he played tennis, then I did too. If he could do 10 pull-ups and 30 sit ups, I was determined to do the same. Sports were very important in our family...football, baseball, hockey. My brother excelled at it all and I followed suit. When it came to school and my education, I was also extremely motivated and worked long and hard to excel there also.

Dad always told us to follow our passion and that true success was the ability to earn a living doing that about which you are passionate. It becomes confusing when you are passionate about many different things. It takes a while to focus on your true calling and filter out your lesser passions. You just have to figure out how to combine all your dreams and create your answer.

I always loved tennis, working out, fitness, art, music, cooking and business. I wasn't like many of my friends who knew early on what field they wanted to pursue.

I started playing tennis at a very early age. Maybe I was 6 or 7 years old. After a couple of years my tennis coach suggested that I start lifting weights. (This is a natural progression. You must work out to balance your body because tennis is a very "one sided" sport.)

I loved the weightlifting so much so that many years later I eventually became a Personal Trainer, which propelled me towards my certifications in aerobics, kickboxing, spinning, pilates, kettlebells, and pre and post-natal fitness. After many years of working out, I found that although I enjoyed it immensely, I was frustrated by the lack of fitness gloves on the market for women. Constantly I was searching for a glove that was not only protective and effective, but fashionable as well.

In college I still played tennis and still worked out and was still frustrated with my hand/glove situation. After graduating from college I worked in investment banking for a short time and then returned to school for my MBA.

One day while visiting my parents in Connecticut, I was complaining to my mother about my hands and the fact that I can't ever find a decent pair of workout gloves. She turned to me and said that I had been whining about that very fact for over 20 years and to stop complaining and do something about it.

That was the beginning of a company called g-loves (www.g-loves.com). I eventually moved to Los Angeles and began shopping for a seamstress. After meeting many naysayers and refusing to listen to their negative chatter, I began the research and development process, giving birth to my first prototype pair of g-loves in 2011.

When I bumped into a friend and told him that I have my prototype made, he dared me to sell 50 pairs within one month. I walked away from that meeting somewhat energized and somewhat frightened. I wondered if I could do it. Five weeks later I had orders for 75 pairs of gloves and was secretly giddy over my business endeavor.

Dreams take time to manifest. I live my passion every day. Someone very wise once said: When you love your job you never work a day in your life. I am a firm believer in putting my dreams out into the universe. This has worked for me.

Hedda Royce
I'm the president and designer of G-Loves.

Stay Driven & Focus on Your Dreams & Goals
by Heather Shanholtz

In life everyone has dreams and goals and a lot of times we have bumps in the road that seem to put a hold on our accomplishments and what we want out of life.

The number one thing you need to do is figure out exactly what you really want out of work, relationships and life's major events first. Stay focused on exactly what you want. No matter how old or young you are, you have to always realize that it is never too late to go after what you want and what you deserve. When planning your goals and dreams remember to set realistic yet challenging ones. Make your goal big enough but not too big to where you hesitate to take that first step.

I'm a big believer in karma, surrounding yourself around positive influential people in your life and also inspiring others to always do better. If you surround yourself with a bunch of deadbeats then you will also be classified as one and probably are one without even realizing it. Always do things to help inspire others and it does make you feel better about yourself and that is where I believe karma truly comes into play. You also have to realize that sometimes bad things happen just so better things can come along even though you may not realize it at the time.

You should always have goals in your life and something to always be working on to better yourself. If not you could find yourself bored, lost and in bad situations. It's okay to change your goals because as life goes on you will also change. Life begins to feel meaningless if you don't have a specific set of goals for yourself. Try writing a list of all of the things you want to accomplish whether it be starting a diet, hitting the gym, going after your dream job and even marriage and a family of your own. Be sure to describe and define your goals. Try to think about how it would feel once you accomplish it and figure out exactly what it would take and the steps to get there. Also write down your personal strengths and the things you need to work on. Always plan ahead and try to give yourself deadlines to meet. Do lots of research on your specific type of goal. There are so many informative websites out there that you can look to for help and advice. Be positive and have belief in yourself. Stay dedicated and motivated to accomplish your list one by one. Dreams and goals are not accomplished overnight and take a lot of willpower so you always have to remember that. The second you reach a goal create another one for yourself. As your goal becomes clearer and you get closer to it you need to remember why you set the goal for yourself in the first place and take pride in yourself that you have almost obtained it.

Life has many twists and turns and is all about change and you have to be able to change with it and roll with the punches. Learn how to adjust with change in a positive way that will benefit you and the ones you care about. Don't ever look back but grow and move forward as hard as sometimes it may be or seem to be. Tomorrow is always another day to get back into gear if you fall backwards. Reminding yourself that you have that drive that just won't quit will make things a lot easier on yourself. If you are feeling down or have optimism, share your feelings and thoughts with someone you trust. Sometimes all we need is that extra boost from family and loved ones. It's never a good thing to hold in all of your feelings because if you do so they explode in a way you would never mean to, or could even push you off of the deep end. Do something that excites you because if you do, it won't be like work once you get there. If you are doing something you love to do it's not like work yet fun and you will find yourself accomplishing things you have never dreamed of. You'll have to go through many obstacles and it might seem tough but you have to keep trying. If you are feeling unmotivated force yourself to do a little bit at a time. When I'm feeling unmotivated it's normally because I'm not getting enough sun (believe it or not vitamin D is very important), not getting in my workouts and alienating myself from family and friends. Always try to stay busy to keep your motivation going.

Along with chasing dreams come a lot of trial and errors. Learn from your mistakes instead of beating yourself up over them. Everyone makes mistakes becoming successful. Be sure to write down all of the mistakes you make along the way so you can be sure not to repeat them.

Stop procrastinating and just do it! Procrastinating doesn't help you in anyway with anything in life. Force yourself to get out there and start. If you continue to push things off then you aren't getting yourself anywhere or closer to your goals and dreams. Once you start you will wish you had started sooner. You will also realize that it wasn't that hard to begin with, once you get in the swing of things. I find the hardest thing is to start. Once you start and stay focused everything moves forward from there. It's just hard initially to get that momentum started and in gear. Always have that "I know I can attitude."

Most importantly always remember that it is your life and no one controls it but you! Take a hold of everything it has to offer and learn from experiences, always move forward and continue to grow and learn. As long as you're driven, motivated and stay focused on your goals you're going to accomplish anything that you really want to.

Heather Shanholtz
I'm a full time model, talent recruiter, a networker and an all round entrepreneur.

Empowering Women
by Jana Stewart

Growing up in a household with two older brothers, I got the desire to bond with other females at an early age. My brothers were involved in a variety of sports and fitness activities so of course I wanted to do the same. Even when they told me what they were doing was not for girls, I ignored them and did it anyway. As I got older and started participating in activities such as sports, dance, drama, it became evident that when you put a group of like-minded women in a room, amazing things happen. Whether it's sports, business, spiritual, community, we make things happen and encourage each other along the way. This reason alone is why I created the Bikini Booty Club, a sisterhood of women from all walks of life with one common goal: to be healthy in every aspect of their lives.

The Bikini Booty Club is different from any other fitness club, women's group, or organization because we are a well rounded group that not only focuses on health and fitness, but women's empowerment, careers, financial freedom, and overall happiness. Because people in general draw from others for inspiration, our primary objective is to inspire women to live their best lives. Our events are never the same and never typical. They range anywhere from workouts in the park to healthy happy hours, spa trips, financial seminars, and online training and coaching. My passion is health, fitness, and active lifestyle living. Not only do I want women to look and feel good physically, but I want their minds to be right too. Over the years I have watched amazing things happen before, during, and after various fitness events. It's simple - when we look our best, we feel our best, and that builds confidence and self esteem. Those traits carry over into our relationships, businesses, careers, and overall quality of life. When we feel empowered, there's nothing that can stop us. We all need a vessel in which we filter out the negative and filter in the positive. My vessel happens to be health and fitness. I workout daily because that's my time to set the tone for my day, visualize, and get myself revved up to take on the day!

These are the tips that I share with women all over the world to be empowered:

1. Define your "Why" and make it so powerful that there's nothing that can deter you from it. My "why" is my family. In February of 2012 I lost the most important man in the world, my father, Ellis Stewart. He was diagnosed with cancer in the summer of 2011 and passed away less than a year later, almost two weeks before his 77th birthday. That devastating loss not only caused me to focus more on preventive health and putting only the best nutrients into my body, but it also created a sense of urgency for me to put myself in the situation to be able to spend even more quality time with my family. We don't have forever on this planet so what we do with our time is so important. My family is my rock and they keep me going. Everything I do, every obstacle I overcome, and every hour of work I put in each day is for them.

2. Set goals. Not just once a year, but daily, monthly, bi-monthly, yearly. Always be working towards something. Health and fitness goals are so much fun to tackle. When we accomplish them, we can actually "see" the results very clearly. When I set a fitness goal and accomplish it, it makes me soar in other areas of my life. I feel unstoppable, powerful, empowered! If we don't set goals, we have nothing to aim for, nothing to work for, so it becomes easy to lay low, relax, and not have a sense or urgency. That's not how we want to go through life. We must always be reaching higher, wanting to do more, connect with more people, and transform more lives.

3. Find a great network of like-minded women. When I first got

into health and fitness, it was as a figure competitor. I was on a training team and there were about four of us who would train together, grocery shop together, travel and compete together. No matter how we did at our competitions, we all still felt like winners because we were supporting each other and creating our own champion moments. When that group dismantled, I felt alone and not so powerful at all. These days I have a whole team of thousands of women, Bikini Booty Club Fitness. We are located all over the world; we unite on social media and motivate, encourage, and inspire each other. The goals that many of the women are accomplishing are amazing! We talk about business, love, careers - I feel like I have thousands of sisters all over the world. I never feel alone and always feel supported.

4. Dream BIG. Constantly visualize, and listen to something motivational daily. I have a ritual that I do every morning. I meditate, pray, and listen to or read at least 10 minutes of something motivational and inspiring. Sometimes it's spiritual and sometimes it's from a successful entrepreneur or athlete. We have the power to determine the outcome of our days, experiences, and moods. That's why it's crucial to start the day off on a positive note with strong intentions of positive outcomes. What we think about we bring about, and I know that we all want to bring goodness, happiness, and success into our lives daily.

5. Always be active! Whether it's a daily workout or taking the stairs instead of the elevator, any form of exercise will cause us to release endorphins, which can be accompanied by a positive and energizing outlook on life. Getting outdoors is a perfect way to do this. There's something about the fresh air that really clears your mind. It's amazing how a little exercise and fresh air can turn any situation into something much better!

6. Always be humble and grateful. Once we acknowledge that

everything we have comes from a higher power, we realize the importance of being grateful for everything that we have accomplished and done in this world. Staying humble helps us to veer away from developing egos and allows us to receive even greater rewards. Take a moment out of your day to either think about what you are grateful for or give someone a call to let him or her know. Spreading goodness is a great way to brighten someone's day and in turn bring more positive experiences into your life.

7. Be daring and adventurous. If we sit around always waiting for the right moment, life could very well pass us by. We have to be daring, live for the moment, take chances and DARE to go after what we want. This could mean doing something very small like taking a trip alone or something adventurous like climbing Mt. Kilimanjaro. Whatever it is that you dream of doing, whether big or small, just DO IT!!

These are rules that I try my best to follow on a daily basis. Being an entrepreneur is not always easy so I have had to create a template to get me through the many obstacles that have come my way. I have found that bonding with like-minded, powerful women is a sure fire way to keep ourselves uplifted and empower us to be the successes that we were put on this earth to be!

Jana Stewart
I'm a lifestyle transformation coach.

Writing Contracts to Lifting Weights
by Tiffany Upshaw

I always knew I was going to be someone or something great, but I could never find it within myself to know exactly what that something was. When you're young, you always have these high hopes and dreams to go off to college, get your degree, and literally walk off the graduation stage and right into a several figure job, living life happily ever after. Well, in the real world, we all have so many different paths to choose but it's not always about finding something that you like to do, it's finding something that you truly love and have a passion for; it's your calling.

It was 2008 and I was a 21yr. old student at Edison State College, obtaining my Associate in Arts Degree. I was working around my school schedule as a real estate agent for about a year and talk about a tough schedule to balance! I was receiving calls from my clients in the middle of my classes to inquire about visiting properties and anyone who knows the real estate business, knows that when a client wants something, you deliver and make it ASAP! Needless to say, I was doing all that I could to make school and my career work for me and try to remain sane at the same time, but that type of business is 24/7/365 and when money calls, you run!

After nearly working myself overtime, I stayed in school but decided to stop practicing real estate as it was too demanding of me, my time, and my focus. I literally didn't know what else I wanted to do as a career. I thought I had everything all planned out for myself; to continue college and make a great living in real estate and it took me awhile to see exactly what I had a drive to do as my next "career path". I would stay up so many nights just researching careers and did several attempts at different things but nothing seemed of any interest to me until one night, it was just one of those late and desperate nights of researching that my 'calling' fell right into my lap.

It was the days of MySpace, a pretty popular social network at the time and I remember my attention span drifting away from researching and onto my profile page just skimming through my friends profiles until I saw I had a message in my inbox. I clicked on the message, read it, and notice that it had been from a gentleman who worked for the supplement company, Optimum Nutrition & American Bodybuilding, asking if I would be interested in being an Endorsed Athlete & Fitness Model for the company.

Now, after reading it, I instantly thought that it was some random guy just trying to lure me into a fake opportunity especially since I had no experience whatsoever in the fitness/bodybuilding industry, but however did have some modeling experience.

I kindly reply back to him stating that I did have an interest in the opportunity and asked what I needed to do to proceed. He wrote back saying that he would send over a contract, that I should read it over and if I agree to it and still had an interest, to sign it and send it back to him. I printed out the contract, read it and also decided to have my friends mother, who was an attorney, read it and let me know if it was legit. Turns out, that contract was as legit as they come and that was to be my ticket to a whole new beginning!

In October of 2008, I was officially an Endorsed Athlete and Fitness Model with Optimum Nutrition & American Bodybuilding. I was ecstatic but I didn't even know where to start, what to do, or how to represent a fitness supplement company especially with no type of "bodybuilding" physique except for a small 125lbs cheerleader type build that I'd had since high school. I immediately got with a trainer and began to learn and teach myself about nutrition and fitness. I saw the other ladies that were a part of the company and knew that in order to make this a success; I needed a body like the rest of the girls on "Team ON/ABB" and was determined to get it so that I could look and be the part.

It was 2009 and the first year that the NPC (National Physique Committee) had implemented a "Bikini" division for women who wanted that toned and fit look instead of hard muscle. I loved the 'toned bikini' look that they wanted so after months of training and transforming my body into something phenomenal, I decided to enter into the NPC's Bikini division and compete for the first time. Not only did I bring my body to the best shape of my life but I took first place in my class! At this moment it was when I realized that the fitness industry was something that I never knew I could have had a love and passion for, but I did know that I had found something that I could be that 'someone or something great'.

Since then, I've become an entrepreneur and am one of the Co-Founders of The Scoopie; a scoop that has a funnel on the side that eliminates the use for a paper funnels and messes when trying to pour a powdered supplement (protein, baby formula, pre-workout) in a container with a small spout.

It is sold in nutrition stores and gyms within the United States, and is now on Amazon.com! That opportunity back in 2008 has truly changed my life and motivated me to grow to become a staple within the fitness industry.

So you see it's about having patience and accepting good opportunities that come to you. I went from sitting in an office writing contracts, to sitting on a weight bench doing shoulder presses. My passion manifested to me and I found my love for something that has currently brought me great success. I've competed numerous times in the bikini division and am now nationally qualified to compete and become an IFBB Bikini Professional. I am thankful every day that I am a major inspiration to people from all walks of life who want to change their life and their habits for a healthier future.

Tiffany Upshaw
I'm an Optimum Nutrition, team ABB, ProTan endorsed athlete and fitness model. A national level NPC bikini competitor, part of Team Blade and co-founder of The Scoopie.

Acknowledge Your Past, Embrace Your Future
by Deanna Wilson

Philippians 3: 13-14, "Brethren, I do not regard myself as having laid hold of it yet; but one thing I do: forgetting what lies behind and reaching forward to what lies ahead, I press on toward the goal for the prize of the upward call of God in Christ Jesus."

I started F5 Lifestyle a year ago. It began as more of an outlet. I had been posting health and fitness statuses on my social media account and it occurred to me one day that not every one of my friends is into that kind of lifestyle. My husband and I put our heads together and talked about what was most important in my life and what I saw as being most important for a person to live a well-rounded healthy lifestyle. We came up with 5 F's: Faith, Family, Friends, Food, and Fitness. F5 Lifestyle was born. I launched the page on social media and began having fun posting inspirational, motivational, and educational information. But I knew. I KNEW that God had something MORE for F5 Lifestyle. Through the encouragement of friends and by the inspiration of God it is developing and growing even as I write.

I grew up a high school and college athlete and I have been involved in the fitness industry for about 16 years as an aerobics instructor. I have had certifications in almost every area of aerobic exercise but my favorites are Strength Training, Core, and Pilates. I spent some time as a personal trainer and worked 10 years as a physical therapy technician. The study of nutrition has been an ongoing hobby and the connection between what we eat and how our bodies perform became an even greater interest as my children began getting involved in sports.

I am genetically predisposed to obesity. I do not come from a lean stock of people. Diabetes runs strong on my father's side but as I survey both sides of my family, most of the obesity has come from lack of nutrition education and, therefore, improper eating habits. In defense of my family, most of them have NOW educated themselves on good nutrition and keep their weight at healthy levels.

So how does the scripture passage that I started this chapter with have anything to do with any of this? Everything! Here is my story through bullet points.

*My mom and biological father divorced by the time I was 2. I never really saw him again until I met him at 16. I saw him a couple more times until I was 19 and then never saw him again. I found out he died when I was about 26. No one ever told me.

*My mom met and married a man that turned out to be an abusive alcoholic. For 10 years he made our lives a living hell. He only pushed me around a couple of times but he would, almost on a nightly basis, come home drunk and verbally abuse my mom. About half that time he physically abused her. I'll spare you the details of 10 years worth of tragic stories but it all ended one night when I thought he was going to sexually molest me. He left the room for a second and I ran out of our apartment and hid at the neighbours. When my mom returned home it turned into a night of extreme physical abuse for her. He finally left the next morning. Come to find out he had sexually molested several of his nieces so my fear was not unwarranted. He died alone in a government assisted care facility in another state crippled and unable to communicate due to so much brain damage from alcohol.

*I was sexually molested by several family members of that man's family.

*By the time I was 16 my single parent mom worked 2-3 jobs to make sure my younger brother and I had everything we needed. That left me alone a lot when I wasn't playing sports. I started dating and ended up getting pregnant. I determined that I was not going to have a baby and ended his/her life through abortion. I'm thankful for God's forgiveness and grace and I am comforted that I will see my child one day in heaven.

I had already prayed to receive Jesus Christ as my Lord and Savior when I was 14. My mom, brother, and I had, at one time, secretly moved away from the abuser and it just so happened that our apartment was right behind a little church. I changed schools and found a friend that attended that church and invited me to the youth group Bible study one night. I was already VERY aware of God. As far back as I can remember I just KNEW there was a God. Although I knew Jesus was my Savior I was still so immature and already carried so much baggage that I made bad choices and, therefore, my pregnancy when I was 16. So what's the point of all this?

The point is that tragedy happens. While we are on this earth we will experience death, sickness, disaster, abuse, etc. It was never God's intention for us to live this way but because of Adam's sin we are now subject to anything and everything this world and people throw at us. What are we to do? Are we to live with the victim mentality? Are we going to let tragic circumstances now define us? Are we going to let the actions of others toward us dictate our own personal choices now? NO!

Look at the scripture again. Paul says, "...forgetting what lies behind...". It's time to let our pasts go. It's time to quit using it as an excuse for unhealthy behavior. It's time to quit letting it define who we are today. But why is it so important to let go of the past? Because God has SO MUCH MORE FOR US and we can't embrace our future if we have our arms wrapped around the past!

If we look at the scripture passage again and go back a few verses Paul says, "I count all things loss in view of the surpassing value of knowing Christ Jesus my Lord, for whom I have suffered the loss of all things, and count them rubbish in order that I may gain Christ, and be found in Him". (vs. 7-9). Paul has a lot to boast about as far as his pedigree. But he ALSO was a persecutor of the church. He was the one holding all the cloaks when the first martyr of the Christian church was stoned! Paul ordered the arrest, imprisonment, and death of countless Christians because he considered it his duty!

Friends, Paul considered his pedigree and his persecution nothing but garbage compared to his knowing Jesus Christ! He let it go! He could have, and probably did at some point, grieve over his own actions and the commands he gave to kill Christians. But he didn't dwell in his past because he looked toward his future! He was going to, "press on toward the goal for the prize of the upward call of God in Christ Jesus" (vs. 14).

You and I have a calling on our lives. It is to KNOW Jesus Christ (John 3:16) and then it is to LOVE GOD and LOVE OTHERS (Matt.22:37-38). I submit that when we KNOW Jesus Christ and realize that He has the most exciting and fulfilling plan for our lives, we no longer want or need to hold onto our past. Like Paul, we can say, it's "rubbish". My past is my past. Your past is your past. It is what it is. People hurt us and we hurt others. Now is the time to let go of what lies behind and reach forward. It's time to stop using food or alcohol to self medicate the pain in our hearts and allow the Great Physician to heal what only He can heal.

For me, personally, one of the greatest ways that I can LOVE God and LOVE others is by taking care of myself. That means that I am purposeful about what I eat, drink, how much I sleep, and how much I exercise. I want to honor God by respecting this one body that He has entrusted to me. Then, I can be the best wife, mother, daughter, sister, aunt, friend, but most importantly, Servant of God. I challenge you to do the same!

Because of Jesus Christ, I have been married for 27 years to my husband, Mike, who has been a pastor and is currently serving as a State Senator. We have 3 children, our son, Sam, and two daughters, Grace and Jessie, all of whom have an understanding of the importance of fitness and nutrition as it relates to God and others.

It's time. Let it go.

Acknowledge Your Past. Embrace Your Future!

Deanna Wilson
I'm a wife, mother and woman of God, wanting to make a difference in the lives of others through the F5 Lifestyle.

What is Success? How is it Measured?
by Jenn Zerling

What does it mean to be successful? How do we measure success? It isn't tangible, so how do we know we achieved it? Gosh, just when we view the guy or gal next door as a very successful person, we find out later that he or she wasn't as successful as we first thought. How is this possible; I always wondered.

As I go through life, I realize more and more that success is something that we each determine on our own. The most successful people in life aren't the ones who make a certain dollar amount each year, rather, they are the ones who find joy in every day, and in the things they do, including their work. Successful people are the ones who balance work and play, keep their bodies and minds fit and feel ready whenever a task is presented to them. This person doesn't stress about money, rather (s)he thinks about ways to earn it. This person never stresses about deadlines or obligations to family, rather (s)he practices good time management skills. This person never sees work as work, rather (s)he feels like the job is a conduit of self expression.

Being successful is an attainable state of being no matter who you are and what you do. I am realizing this more and more every day. This is what I find joy in teaching to others. In fact, my success as a fitness expert, isn't in the number of clients I train or the amount of wellness programs I run. My success is measured on how well my teachings are received by my "students" and how well they do with my plan. My goal is to teach people how to reach a state of self actualization, the ability to fulfill your potential and become all that you are capable of becoming. When my students/clients lose weight (from fat not muscle) and claim a state of self actualization, my heart explodes with joy like fireworks on the

4th of July. I thrive on knowing that I am able to provide the appropriate tools for individuals to effectively shift their lifestyle so that they can ultimately achieve a healthy way of life.

As I realized my gift of compassion for people who struggle toward optimum health, I began expanding my personal training business to include more hands on education. My master's degree in Kinesiology concluded with a thesis which yielded a successful "Fitness for 30 Minutes" interval program for kids. I've presented this program to physical education teachers around the nation at the American Alliance of Health Physical Education Recreation and Dance (AAHPERD) conferences. In addition, I am teaching physicians how to motivate unmotivated patients at the Age Management Medical Group (AAMG) conference. My goal with these two national conferences was to show teachers and practitioners how to take coaching, training or guidance to the next level for those they come in contact with. I believe in sharing my success with others so that they too can be successful with the people they work with.

My journey has crossed paths with many influential people that I have had the pleasure of diving into conversations that stimulated and continue to stimulate my expertise in areas that I never imagined. For example, if you had asked me 5 years ago about writing a book, I wouldn't have even thought of it as a possibility. However, on my way to a conference in 2010, I had the chance to meet an author who convinced me that I would write not one, but several books. I told him that it would be so neat if I can create a toolbox of strategies for change that can be used throughout a weight loss journey. I wanted to expand my voice beyond the boundaries of my geographic allowing individuals the opportunity to own a good lifestyle adjustment workbook. Breaking the Chains of Obesity, 107 Tools was born in March 2011. The title comes from my beautiful mother who told me she was proud of my accomplishments and success. Coping with her own overweight struggles virtually her entire life, she told me that I am the first generation in our family to have broken the habits or chains of what has been a perpetual cycle of obesity for generations. Hence, Breaking the Chains of Obesity! Mom read my book and lost 35 pounds. While she has not yet arrived at her goal, she has incorporated many of the fundamentals that she learned from the book into her life. This is indicative of true success.

Corporate wellness programs are increasing as a result of healthcare reforms. For this reason, I have formulated a program for corporations which include my coaching, training, and the use of Breaking the Chains of Obesity, 107 Tools as my premier workbook. The true success of a corporate wellness program is seeing transformation in the employees, and more so with the leaders of the company. My work with South Bay BMW in California is proof that when the leaders are on board with healthy lifestyle behaviors, the rest of the team will follow, or eventually become influenced to join in. Since most staff spend between eight to ten hours per day at BMW, it was important to establish a healthy work environment that allows them opportunities for success in their weight loss journeys. As soon as I enter their building, my focus is on attending to the needs of each employee I come in contact with, from start to finish of each session. As a result of their successes with this corporate wellness program, they think clearer, feel better, look better, and are more tolerant of the day to day challenges of the business. Experiencing their successes validates my own success.

Publishing my book, has inspired me to expand into additional writing opportunities. I am now credited for writing for national publications, and developed my own blog www.jzfitness.com.

I'm also a member of two not-for-profit organizations; The American Diabetes Association (ADA) and Matthew Mcconaughey's JK Livin program. These two venues allow me continued success as a humanitarian. My time is spent with the ADA as a lecturer on fitness and nutrition for people who live with diabetes. For JK Livin, I was hired on to share my fitness expertise with high school students in their afterschool program. This is very rewarding work. All of the JK Livin staff utilizes Breaking the Chains of Obesity, 107 Tools as part of their afterschool program curriculum.

The bottom line is this: you must possess passion for what you do in order to be successful. My passion to help people allows me to think outside of the box and bring things from good to great. You can't fake what I do. You either love it or you don't. If I wasn't passionate about helping people, then there is no way I can transfer my energy to another person and add to their success. Patience, persistence and perseverance, along with passion and compassion are what make JZ successful.

Jenn Zerling
I'm the Author of Breaking the Chains of Obesity, 107 tools, fitness expert, national presenter, former captain of Varsity cheerleading, and a very lovable girl!

VOLUME IV - FIND BALANCE

Motherhood
by Alli Breen

Motherhood - it's a sport. 24/7, 365 days a year, whether your children are next to you or across the globe you are always on call. At times it is all consuming and extremely overwhelming. I believe that, for women who choose to be mothers, it is the most challenging and rewarding job on the planet!

A child's first role model is often their mother. A mother's mood can affect her children on a daily basis and her actions can impact them for a lifetime. So how can we set our children up for success though our day-to-day life and actions? We can do this through leading by example! One of the best rewards of being a healthy, fit mom is seeing your kids take notice and then enjoy leading a healthy lifestyle in the same manner in which you have demonstrated to them.

Most mothers want one simple thing for their children - health. Overall thriving mental and physical health. How can we as women help our children achieve this? By taking the best care of ourselves on every level that we can control. And the only thing you truly can control is yourself.

Demonstrating a healthy lifestyle through your speech, actions, postures, boundaries, nutrition and exercise all play a role in how your kids learn to interact with others and in developing the confidence they feel within themselves. If you are happy and feel great so will your children, think of them as a mirror.

Leading by example can start at any minute of any day, so if you are new to taking charge of your health or needing to fine-tune a few things, remember the importance of the present moment because it's all you have. Your past does not equal who you are, now or in the future! Use positive thinking and visualization as a way to feel like your dream self as a woman and a mother.

My Top 5 Health Tips That Will Make You a Happy Healthy Mom:

1. Nutrition: Motherhood is a sport, so eat like an athlete. Nutrition can make or break you mentally, emotionally and physically.

Eating vitamin-rich foods every few hours throughout the day is essential for getting results you want - high energy levels, a great body, glowing skin, and a great attitude. Try getting your kids in the kitchen with you to help out with healthy, quick recipes and they will soon be eating things you thought they would never touch!

2. Exercise: Nothing can change a mood faster than a workout! Moving your body 4-6 days a week for 30 to 60 min is the best way to increase daily energy and overall strength and endurance for the demands of motherhood. Taking time for good nutrition and workouts should be a non-negotiable part of your life, like a business meeting you cannot miss.

Hygiene: Brush and floss those pearly whites. Exfoliate and moisturize head to toe, and shape those nails! I personally do my nails one day a week and scrub under them daily, whether they are painted or not.

3. Fashion: No matter the size on your clothing label, wear clothes and accessories that make you feel good. Pick the colors and styles that make you feel comfortable yet confident!

4. Music: Positive music can change the way you feel instantly. I have music playing around me 90% of the time! Music can be so inspiring and uplifting, and sharing fun and happy music with kids will build memories that when heard will last a lifetime, so get those playlists pumping!

5. Lastly my bonus tip is to get enough sleep, which depending where you are on your motherhood journey is a bit more difficult. Try to get eight hours within a 24-hour period even if broken up. Being rested will

help control moods, appetite, and energy levels.

Incorporating these tips will change your life and make you the best version of you. Ladies, it's never too late, and with these tips and the right attitude anything is possible!

Life is short - you only have a few years that you can push your baby in a stroller, or get on the jungle gym with them so don't sit on the sidelines, get in the game and have fun!

So remember one thing ladies, if you want to have a healthy family; start today, because as I always say, "Today is Your Tomorrow."

Alli Breen

I focus on instructing, coaching, motivating & inspiring others to take their health, healing & happiness to the next level.

Trust in the Process
by Rita Catolino

Don't rush to the end; you may realize you have missed the most important part!

Having been through my own personal physical transformation has really defined who I am today. If it weren't for the struggles and hurdles I was forced to face, I wouldn't have the privilege of helping other women see and develop their own true potential and optimal selves.

A body transformation is so much more than just physical. It affects so many levels of our being, including our mental, emotional and physical states. There are many layers of the "onion" that make up our journey. My experience has shown that one of the biggest issues that women face when they embark on a fat loss journey is the fixation on the outcome; the number on the scale. An extreme focus on that tangible number makes so many of us miss what could be the best part of the process, the meat of the sandwich if you will, the journey itself.

When someone decides that they have reached the breaking point with regard to their body image – that moment when they decide this is the limit, some plan of action is usually quick to follow. Often the plan comes when we are at the height of frustration. Usually the plan includes some or all of the following: the detox, cleanse, 21 day juicing, lifting weights, the spin classes or the weekly boot camps usually become the areas of focus for the next few months. The cupboards get cleaned, the junk food tossed and the social calendar gets put on hold. Sound familiar??

But what about the daily encounters with the scale, or as I like to call it: the "kill-my-mood-machine?" Our initial new focus, which was a healthy one, may easily be taken over by the number on the scale and may even become an obsession. "I will not give up." "I will not stop until the number says x etc., etc." I have encountered much of this behaviour first-hand, and sadly when I started on my own journey, I too was guilty of the same focus.

The good news is that I learned quite early on that this was no way to live my life. I had a family, friends and a healthy body. But I was comparing myself to a number - a subjective standard of what I thought was my ticket to happiness. It was not until I threw out my "perfectionist" standards - along with the scale - that I began to live my own journey of success and actually enjoyed each and every step along the way.

Here's how the shift changed from scale-focus to more life-focus. Let's start with the gym. My training sessions which started off as a means to an end - my ticket to "skinny" - were completed with little thought and as quickly as possible so I could run home and tick it off the list. I was just one workout closer to the new me. Now, however, after more than 6 years on my health and wellness path, I have realised that training is one of the most enjoyable parts of my day. I no longer look at it as thing on the list, but more like a special hour where I dedicate movement, flexibility, agility, strength and power to the body. Wow. Who doesn't deserve that? I also realised that when I stopped to look around, I was surrounded by people with similar stories and goals, all getting their daily dose of endorphins right alongside me. Conversations were had, tips were shared, and the gym not only became a place to create my new body temple, but also a place for social encounters.

Once I got hooked on the training, I knew that the food improvements had to follow. Let's face it, wine every weekend and enormous helpings of bread, pasta and cheese were not helping me achieve my goal. So why not cut it all out, and live on green tea and vegetables smoothies for 3 months? Well, lucky for me, I love food way too much to throw away any opportunity given to use my pearly whites. Let's face it; our teeth were given to us not only to smile, but to CHEW our food!! I was not going to ignore that fact. So although at the beginning I was using extreme methods of restriction to get me to my goal (the number on the scale) as fast as possible, I soon realised that I was NOT happy in the process. How many of you use this method?

What good is it to be in size 4 skinny jeans if I wasn't happy and my hair, skin, nails and sex drive were more than dead? Once again, listening to my body and the messages it was giving me, made me wake up and smell the coffee, or in my case the food! I decided to not overly restrict myself, nor go back to my former ways of daily pasta bowls and hunks of cheese. Rather, my success and sustainability over the past 6 years have been thanks to moderation, balance and enjoying every moment along the way.

My version of moderation is now 1 glass of red wine with my family on the weekends instead of 1 bottle. I enjoy vacations without scales, family gatherings for the people, not the food, and ice cream with my daughter on a warm summer day - not a whole liter alone at midnight by the open freezer door. I have learned to love my life, my progress and most importantly my journey. I hope you can start to write your own rules to your journey and celebrate your success along your path.

Cheers!

Rita Catolino

I'm a certified personal trainer, online coach, motivational speaker, fitness writer & cover model. My passion for fitness & helping others comes from having gone through many of my own struggles with weight my entire life.

Finding Balance & Loving Yourself
by Kattie Fleece

As a mommy of two, sometimes it can be hard to juggle all of the things that come my way. Between activities, sports, work, meal prepping, bath time, workouts, etc. it can be a bit overwhelming. Any mother can relate. In fact, any NON-mother can relate. We tend to get so busy wrapped up in everything going on around us that we often forget to take care of ourselves.

HOW DO I DO IT? One of the main things that I've learned throughout the years is to be a good TIME MANAGER. To-do lists have become my best friend. I'm sure you've heard the statement, "I don't have time, I MAKE time". How true that is. One of the things that is always on my list of things to do is "workout". That might mean getting up at the crack of dawn before the kids wake up and before my husband leaves for work to squeeze in a workout. Or it might mean that I have to workout on my lunch break. I just make sure it gets done. So often, it's easy to feel guilty for leaving your children to take time for YOU. But, then you've got to think of WHY you are taking care of yourself in the first place. I know for me personally, it's because of my children. They are my WHY. I want to be around for them as long as I can and be able to keep up with them.

Another tip that I've found helpful for someone who is trying to live a fit life is MEAL PLANNING. If you fail to plan, plan to fail. How often do we forget to lay something out for dinner, so we end up running through the McDonald's drive through.... again. I'm guilty of it, that's for sure. When you can plan for the week, it's much easier to stay on track with your goals. This will also help with time management. If you have a plan of attack and are able to prep your meals earlier in the week, this will save a lot of time and headaches when it's time to eat. Often enough, I notice when I'm slacking, so does my family. They count on me to lead them in a healthy lifestyle.

SET GOALS. Whether they are long term goals or small weekly goals, having a goal in mind will help you strive for something. I encourage you to write them down and put them some place where you will see them every day (i.e. bathroom mirror, refrigerator, dashboard of your car, etc.). Even if your goal is to drink more water for the week, it is something for you to work towards. I know that this has helped me tremendously in the past. My mother recently told me that if you do not have goals set in life, then you will hit your target every time - which is nothing.

And lastly, LOVE YOURSELF. Realize that YOU are enough. No matter what you may be going through, taking the time to LOVE yourself is crucial. This goes back to what I said earlier about taking time for YOU. In today's world, it is so easy to get caught up in comparing yourself to everyone else.

You might look at the cover of a magazine and think to yourself "I will never look like that" or listen to the media call your favorite celebrity "fat" when you would love to be her size. Listen, the only person you should be competing with is YOURSELF. Strive to be the best version of YOU possible. If you can do that, then you've done your job.

One of my favorite Bible verses clearly teaches us to take care of the body God has given us. In Corinthians 6:19-20 it says "Do you not know that your body is a temple of the Holy Spirit within you, whom you have from God, and that you are not your own? For you have been purchased at a price. Therefore, glorify God in your body.".

In everything that we do, we must glorify HIM in our bodies. We have ONE chance to treat our bodies like the temples that they are. In Proverbs 31, we are reminded again the importance of training and our purpose for it. "She sets about her work vigorously; her arms are strong for her tasks.".

Every time I lack motivation, I remind myself of these verses. Will it be easy? No. Will it be worth it? Absolutely.

BELIEVE and you will ACHIEVE!

Kattie Fleece
I'm a Certified Personal Trainer, Group Fitness Instructor and Pilates Coach.

My Life, My Puzzle
by Rose Gracie

It's very surreal that as I look back at my life I come to the most insane realization that the pieces will always come together at the end and everything just makes a lot of sense.

I was always very fortunate, very loved, and grew up with quite a bit in Rio de Janeiro. I was always surrounded by friends and family and the variety of life that comes with having such a large family. One of my grandfathers, Carlos Imperial, was a politician, artist, producer, musician, actor, TV personality and anything else he wanted to be in Brazil. He was, without a doubt, one of the biggest influences in my life if not the biggest.

My Grandfather Carlos never put limits on what could be accomplished. He always made it very clear that if either my sister or I ever wanted something we could just go out and get it. It was just that simple. It was so simple, in fact, and so real that to question that fact would be a huge mistake. My grandfather was an extremely well accomplished businessman and although he came from a very wealthy background everything he had was attained with his own hard work and sweat. He was extremely intelligent and a very critical thinker. I remember he would host huge and extravagant parties for the who's who of politics one day and the who's who of TV personalities another day and the who's who of musicians on yet another day. To help get me used to talking to anyone, my grandfather always put me in charge of opening the door and greeting all the guests. He was teaching me how to be ready to talk to anyone no matter who they were and how to get what I wanted or at times what he wanted, as I still remember my script when he would see a beautiful young lady that he would like to get to know a bit more. =)

My mom used to always say to me "Rich grandparents, noble

children, broke grandchildren" in an attempt to make me understand that I needed to work very hard and not count on money lasting forever. I never questioned her quotes. I believed in what she said wholehearted and that gave me a very good work ethic. While I was still very young my mom became the "godmother" of an orphanage in Rio. One day, my mom and I went to meet some of the kids and visit the place where they were staying. When we got there, I was mortified by the conditions that those kids were living in. My mom, like most of the ladies in my family, did not waste anytime and started to make changes in those kid's lives. Inspired by her thoughtfulness, I too wanted to reach out and help in any way that I could. My birthday was coming up and a new theater play was in town. My grandfather bought an entire section of tickets for me to invite my friends. (seriously...who does that? =) My mom suggested to me that we invite some of the kids from the orphanage and I thought that was a great idea. So my mom rented a bus for them so that they could come and watch the play. We reserved the first few rows of seats just for them so they could feel special. I remember that being my favorite present and by far the highlight of my birthday party because those kids were genuinely appreciative of my generosity.

As a kid, some of my weekends were spent with my Grandfather Helio, from my Dad's side of the family. He was a super fun grandpa that always tucked us in at night and always brought us a breakfast smoothie in bed in the morning. His bedtime stories were also the best because he would always fight the bad guy and win! My Grandpa Helio was a wise man and taught me how to shoot a gun when I was about 9 years old. I remember when I was young and my mom was telling my Grandpa Helio about my dance lessons and musical accomplishments and he thought everything was silly. He turned to my mom and said, "The most important lesson she needs to know is that a woman should heat her stomach at the stove and cool it off at the sink.". He honestly believed that the "guys were going to lead the way!" Oh boy, if he only knew. I honestly wish he was here now to see that it took a woman to make some changes to something he loved very deeply and to fix it to his liking with hopes that those changes would keep his legacy alive. I think he would have been very proud of me and for that, I am happy. My Grandpa Helio taught me that nothing in life happens for no reason. As I continue in the journey to uphold his legacy I realize that he was right all along.

I love and have always loved very deeply. I didn't really have a lot of boyfriends, but the ones I did have were always very intense and long lasting relationships. I always had a very deep connection with my partners and I still care for all of them and cheer for them in their lives. My relationships were very healthy and for that I am very grateful. My past relationships taught me that people don't change but their views, goals and dreams do. And when we choose to, at a certain point, walk together on the same path in our lives it doesn't have to be forever. You may one day realize that your roads are going in different directions and that is ok. You can part ways and continue on your journey as friends and that should be something positive.

Being the first of an entire generation for all sides of my family was pretty amazing! I always had a motherly instinct about me; some people are just wired that way I guess. I loved my siblings and younger cousins more than life itself! I was madly in love with them and I couldn't wait to have kids of my own. Someone once told me that when I had my own kids I would love them more then anything and I did not believe it was possible to love more than I already did. But after I had my kids I found out that they were right. The connection that you have with your children is different. It is still amazing to see the kids in my family who have grown up and now having kids of their own. They are having their own moments and forming their own families. Seeing the members of my family mature and grow as individuals has made me realize that the circle of life will continue forever and its a beautiful thing to see.

Nothing happens for no reason. When a friend of mine, who was like a brother to me, invited me to another friend's birthday I really wanted to go, but I was concerned that I probably wasn't going to get any sleep for work the next day. I finally decided that I would only go for less than an hour just to say hi and bye. As I was saying my hello's I all of the sudden noticed this guy walk in. I noticed there was something about him that I was drawn to. He was definitely a leader of his pack and was funny and looked at me very differently than anyone had looked at me before. Even inside of the loud club, I was able to communicate with him as if we were the only two people there. I married Javi a short time later and we have now been married for 8 years. When I said "I do" to him I meant it and knew I was in for the long run. You see marriage is a very difficult thing for everyone and mine was not going to be any different. I have had some major ups, and of course even bigger falls, but when you are really in it for the long run you don't quit. You find solutions. With Javi I learned that as long as there is communication, respect, trust and love we will stay in this path together till death due us part.

Sometimes in life someone will inspire you. Sometimes life will make you think, wonder, dream, and even make you question your senses and beliefs to their core. And as much as you think you know and think that you are prepared, life will surprise you. Nothing, I seriously mean NOTHING, could have ever prepared me for the biggest lesson of my life: motherhood. I have three very different and very amazing daughters that are the center of my world. There is not a day that goes by that I don't think of them and there is not a single thing in this world I wouldn't do for them. They are without a doubt my biggest life lesson and from them

I have learned unconditional love. A love that you can not measure or explain. I just want to make sure I raise them right, to be well adjusted adults that will work hard, that have a good heart, that will love deeply, but will also know when to let go. I want them to always be aware that no matter what they can accomplish anything and they should never be afraid to question everything.

I was very fortunate to be around so many phenomenal people in this life path and I can see clearly now, more than ever, that life is just a big puzzle. With all my experiences and life lessons I have been able to become wiser and obviously completely insane because I truly believe that I can change anything I want in this world.

You see the cycle of life doesn't stop it just takes turns like a winding road down the generations. You must learn to respect that force and accept it for whatever it gives to you. All my relationships and life lessons were very important in molding me, but none of them defined me.

At the end you must understand that what really matters in life is the relationship you have with yourself and that "Life doesn't happen to you, life happens for you.".

Rose Gracie
I'm the woman behind the Gracie Nationals and Gracie World Championships, a mother of 3, dedicating my life to making a positive change in other people's lives.

How to Release Your Inner Zen
by Tara Milhem

"You cannot always control what goes on outside. But you can always control what goes on inside."

Peace and quiet. Aaah.. In the midst of the craziness of the world you might be wondering where people actually find that balance and manage to appear so "zen". Hold tight because you are about to experience it yourself.

How?

No matter what part of the world you are in, whether you are in an ashram in India or in the center of New York City, the ability to silence your mind comes from within. Yes that means everyone, including you, has the ability to do it. Some people call it meditation, some call it consciousness, others call it crazy. Being able to sit with yourself in pure silence is a vital part of self-acceptance. Without mastering this skill, one will always look towards outside sources for happiness.

Take a second to forget your environment and focus entirely on yourself. The following exercise I've designed is going to help you become more present and leave the noise of the world behind. The first time you practice this exercise may feel uncomfortable, but if you dedicate yourself to this practice once a day you will begin to create a balance inside your mind that will clear your head and leave you feeling zen in no time.

Let's begin.

Come into a comfortable seated position in a quiet room. You can cross your legs on the floor, lounge back on your sofa, or sit in any other position that allows your body to relax.

Drown out the noise beyond your control and put these few minutes aside to focus on yourself and your breath. On each inhale envision that you are taking in positive energy in the form of light and on each exhale you are releasing tension, anxiety, and darkness. This practice of visualization will make the meditation more comfortable.

Take a deep breath in through your nose and hold it for 3 seconds. Hold, hold, hold.

Exhale out through your nose keeping your mouth closed.

Repeat that breath slowly 2 more times. Eyes closed and shoulders relaxed.

Become aware of your toes beginning to numb and your mind wandering in every other direction. Rather than shunning your thoughts, welcome and accept them. It is normal to have thoughts, but don't let them take you out of your practice. Simply acknowledge their presence and continue with the breath. By returning to your breath whenever your mind wanders away, you are creating a safe space for your thoughts to reside and stillness to come.

For the next few breaths, follow the simple method outlined below. On each inhale, silently repeat the words "I am" and on each exhale, repeat the word "Calm", then "Relaxed", then "Balanced". Close your eyes and begin.

Breath 1: Inhale "I am", Exhale "Calm"

Breath 2: Inhale "I am", Exhale "Relaxed"

Breath 3: Inhale "I am", Exhale "Balanced"

Repeat 1-3x, or as desired.

Place your hands at your heart in prayer pose, close your eyes, and remind yourself of why you are searching for the zen inside of you. Do you want to release accumulated stress? Improve your health? Increase your memory? Whatever your goals may be, constantly remind yourself of them to keep you on a healthy path for your practice.

Now bring your awareness back to your body and begin to move your toes and your fingers. Stretch your neck side to side. Shake your legs out.

Acknowledge that there is no rush to reach any specific point. Peace of mind is not about reaching a destination; it is the journey that will lead you to your eternal bliss.

Namaste!

Tara Milhem
I'm a wellness designer and the founder of SkinnybyTara, an online community designed to empower and inspire women to live their healthiest lives.

Blessed
by Mary Schmitt

Sweat trickles down my goose-bump covered body as I make my way with agile speed through the gym. My body is undoubtedly pumping with endorphins; it reminds once again why I love this fitness thing so much. Anyone that knows me will tell you that I'm somewhat of an extremist when it comes to training. I train to intensity in the double digits weekly. As I walk through the gym, high on endorphins from my workout; it makes me acknowledge a period of time in my life when training felt forced. As a Health and Wellness Coach it has become apparent to me that many people struggle with these same issues; finding balance. Working out shouldn't be a chore, or a place that we seek superficial comfort. I believe what shifted my perception was a personal experience I had a few years ago; some might think it insignificant... but to me it was a life lesson, and something I will never forget.

In the beginning I never enjoyed my two a day gym trips... and as I dedicated myself more and more to my body; I found that it was something I craved. I craved it for all of the wrong reasons... I became obsessed with having a "perfect body". My motives for working out and dieting were completely aesthetic. I never really noticed my obsession until there were times that it wasn't feasible for me to make it twice, and the absence of my passion would wear on me.

At one point that was not the case... it happens to the best of us. If you are an avid weight trainer you know that the majority of staying with a strict diet and training regimen is a head game, as are most things in life. Perception is everything! A few years ago, on a cold Denver winter night; my entire life changed. Many people would find my story less than an eventful... but to me it was a turning point in consciousness, a moment of extreme clarity and compassion.

I slumped up the stairs with fainting energy, and reached for some workout clothes from my closet… not paying any attention to what I had grabbed. I dressed myself, and went through my usual routine: One gym towel, check… one charged MP3, check… water bottle, check… then into the garage, and out into the late night.

I arrived at the barren gym and walked to my favorite piece of cardio equipment with heavy feet. As I pedaled away, I started contemplating barter in my head… "Okay, so I'm supposed to burn 750 calories during this cardio session, but if I work out on my day off it will be okay if I only burn 500.". Is any of this sounding familiar? As I'm bartering in my head, I take notice to the television screen ahead. There is a woman missing part of her face in a hospital room wheelchair, holding a small child. The image undoubtedly startled me, and to say the least grabbed my attention. I started reading the captions running across the bottom of the screen, and although I started reading late into the story I was able to pick up a message and perhaps a very important lesson.

The woman in the show had mentioned something about being grateful to be there for her daughter, regardless of having to live the rest of her life with remnants of her face left behind and sitting in a wheelchair. It was hard for me to keep tears away, especially in my tired fragile state. The woman was more than elated, and you could truly feel her sense of joy.

The story documenting the woman's unfortunate situation made me realize something that I had obviously forgotten. I glanced down at my legs… moving in rhythmic harmony with my arms, perfectly even and balanced, throbbing with power. I quickened my pace, and could feel my heart pumping with adrenaline and my lungs taking in the Colorado air with ease. It occurred to me that I had forgotten how truly blessed I am… two arms, two legs, two lungs, a heart, and every opportunity in the world to succeed… There I was feeling sorry for myself; more worried about abs than my health. I was finding excuses why I didn't want to work out…when some didn't have the luxury.

This isn't a story that hasn't been told before. "There's starving kids in Africa." as you sat at a table as a child pushing tuna casserole around with your fork. As if eating your parents' food would actually save starving children in Africa. This story goes deeper than the wives tales of your childhood. Sometimes you need to change your perception on a situation.

That night in the gym I had one of the best cardio sessions of my life. I pushed my able body to the limits, and left that gym soaking wet, feeling accomplished and blessed. I no longer cared so much about having a "perfect body". I began to enjoy the process; the process of improving my health and truly feeling my workouts, presently and earnestly.

My training and diet regimen was no longer a race to the finish line, it was a gift to be enjoyed. I believe the lesson I learned here was that sometimes we need to take a step back and acknowledge how we are perceiving situations.

The next time you are lacing up your tennis shoes wishing you were on your couch, take a second to remember that you are blessed.

Mary Schmitt
I'm a Health and Wellness Coach and the creator of The Total Body Transformation.

Superwoman; Fact or Fiction?
by Nicole Sims

I don't know how she does it? This woman, who had a face of a Cover Girl model, a body out of a fitness magazine, 2 kids (a boy and a girl, of course, both in the gifted program), a high earning job and a housework loving husband who is just a fabulous as she and happens to worship the ground she walks on. Oh, did I mention that she has an amazing social life and is frequently invited to the hottest places around from coast to coast? Sounds too good to be true, right? Well surely there must be some truth to this woman. She has to exist somewhere. I know I've seen her before. Maybe it was on that Reality TV show, you know, the one with the wealthy women with tons of drama? Or maybe I saw her life being documented everyday on my Facebook Feed?

The real truth is she doesn't exist. How do I know? Because I tried my own version of "having it all" and failed miserably.

We have been told that life is about 'balance' and to be a successful and happy woman then that is what we must strive for. Let's say that life was divided into 4 major groups: Family, Self, Work, and Play. For the purpose of this exercise, 'Self' will represent anything that does not have a direct effect on anyone other than you. If we balance correctly, that would allow us ¼ or 25% of our time to focus on each component. Perfect, we just achieved total balance. But wait! Something doesn't go as you planned. Your kid just got sick, you had leave work early (guess you'll have to miss that noon workout too), your boss used that snafu to pass you over for a promotion (she wanted someone more committed to the work), not to mention that you and were husband were counting on that extra income to pay down your student loans to get a better interest rate for you home mortgage, now he is going to have work a second shift. And seemingly overnight, the scales have shifted and what was once this perfectly divided pie now resembles something that exploded in the microwave.

In my own life, I had a period where all I wanted to do or think about was competing on a fitness stage. I thought that this goal of mine would somehow make me feel accomplished. The grueling, intense workouts and strict diet were very consuming. In the beginning, it was very difficult to manage it all. I would actually cook my food on an almost daily basis while also trying to provide an entirely separate meal for my family. My workouts, as well as the commute to the gym easily took up to 3 hours of my day, leaving me exhausted by the end of the night (my husband did not appreciate this side effect). I was just hoping that I could muster up enough energy to do it all over again the next day. This rat race barely left me with energy to spend quality time with my family or friends. Not only was I suffering, but the people that mattered most to me were also suffering.

I had to go back to the drawing board. I had to find out what would work for ME. I learned and most of all ACCEPTED that there were some things that I would have to sacrifice. I would have to let go of perfectionism, embrace vulnerability and simply live in each moment. I learned that it is almost impossible for me to keep my disciplined gym schedule when my kids are out of school (I'm a full-time mom of 3), I also learned that it was essential to precook several days' worth of food needed for my diet in order to follow it.

But most of all I discovered that I didn't need to have extraordinary moments to find happiness because as long as I am aware of my blessings and practice gratitude then true happiness is right in front of me.

Miriam Khalladi

Nicole Sims

I'm an IFBB Figure Pro based out of Seattle, WA. I received my Pro status in 2012 by winning the Overall Figure title at the NPC Nationals and made my pro debut at the invite only, 25th Anniversary Arnold Classic.

Start; Healthy Lifestyle with Balance
by Dionne Sinclair

I see myself as a role model for coworkers and my clients/patients. By making physical activity and healthy eating a priority, I feel I am better able to meet the demands of my job as Manager of the Inpatient Mental Health unit at Toronto's Humber River Hospital.

Growing up, I was a track and field athlete in high school but drifted away from sport and eating the right foods after I became a nurse and a parent. Shift work made it even more difficult for me to watch my diet and have the time to work out. As I was approaching 40 years old I decided it was time to lose the weight I had gained while pregnant with my third child and to rejoin the fitness world.

It was not easy to be disciplined and I worked hard at it. I believe when you stay active, you look good, you feel good and you have more energy on the job to deal with stresses that come up. I believe it is incumbent on all working women to pursue healthy lifestyles, for their own benefit and the benefit of their families. I believe it's important to be fit and able to manage any kind of situation. When you get confronted with multiple of life's stressors, its important to have the energy and endurance to handle all of what life throws at you.

Living a healthy lifestyle is part of my health teaching to patients, friends and families. I like to think I am leading by example. If someone sees me taking the stairs instead of the elevator, they may want to do it, too.

My simple plan I provide for all of the people who ask me how to start on the road to a healthier sustainable lifestyle is visit my "Dionne Sinclair Fitness Model" Facebook Page and hit LIKE, then:

1. Start by doing 1 thing a week and adding a new thing every week;

so that one thing may be cut back on the amount of sugar you consume. If you usually have 3 packets of sugar in your coffee of half and half cream with your coffee. Try 2 packets of sugar and 2% milk. It can be that simple. Nothing too drastic. It took you awhile to build the life you are living; it will take awhile to change to a different lifestyle.

2. Write it down and keep track; Get yourself a note pad and a good pen or write on your iPad or iPhone note pad. Write down your goal. "I want to fit into a size 6 from a 10.", "I want to have sex with the lights on.", "I want to look good naked.". Whatever your goal/goals are, write them down. Next write down what you are prepared to do about it. "I will get up early and go for a morning walk.", "I will go to the gym 3 times per week.". Next write down every day what you eat and what you actually do. Did you do what you said you were going to do?

3. Get rid of your scale. Measure your success by how you feel. How you look in your clothes. Do not let the number on a scale affect your progress. I do not own a scale. Are you able to lift heavier, walk farther, stay active longer. Those are true measures of how you are doing.

4. First week stop eating out; start preparing your meals at home. Pack your lunch. Get simple fruits and vegetables from your local farmers market or from the local supermarket. Have the whole family get involved in preparing meals. Keep it simple. Use nuts, seeds, beans, lentils. Google Clean eating recipes. Call your mother, sister or friends for some of their favorite recipes.

5. Second week add 1 glass of water before every meal; you are not hungry, you are thirsty. I believe if you drink the glass of water before you eat. You may find that you were not hungry at all. If you still feel hungry after you drink the water then go ahead, eat your meal. Drink again after the meal. It aids in digestion and cleanse your palate.

6. Third week cut your portions in half. Do not eat everything on

your plate. In North America, portion sizes can be very large. I tell family and friends to make a fist. This shows them the size of their stomach. You do not need more than the size of your fist as a meal portion. Switch to a small bowl or a saucer. The big dinner plates take too much to fill and smaller size plates help you keep the portions small. If it does not fit in the bowl, you do not need it.

7. Fourth week, add more veggies and less starchy foods to your meals; yes, its all about food. Your size is controlled 70% by what you eat. Add more green leafy veggies to your diet. Get rid of processed foods. Clean out your kitchen of foods in boxes processed from factories.

8. Fifth week start walking in the morning and evening; yes only now we are exercising. You can start as early as week one however, I want to show how it's about what you are eating and how much you eat and not exercise alone. Walk, run, jog, bike, skip, go to a gym and walk on one of their cardio machines. Use a treadmill. I believe in slow cardio. Slow speed with a high incline. 2.3-2.5 speed on the treadmill with an incline of 10-15. Try it for 6 weeks. I promise you will see a big difference. Stay on for 40-60 minutes.

9. Sixth week. Add 25 pushups and sit-ups every morning and evening after your walk. You can do this from week one as well. I just want everyone to know that, to live a healthy lifestyle, what you eat is more important. If you belong to a gym, join a fitness class. I teach Body Pump and Zumba. Exercising in a group setting is beneficial. You form a community and it gives you purpose to get there, meet friends and push yourself. No gym, no problem. There are is lot of free information online. Search for workout routines you are interested in.

10. Keep following the page (Dionne Sinclair Fitness Model) for example of exercises, meal suggestions and power moves. Read the motivational posts and see if any apply to your life. It's important to believe

that you can do it. You are not alone. Never ever give up.

Dionne Sinclair

I'm a lightning rod of energy that engages and motivates everyone I meet. Caring, hardworking and driven. I believe everyone can live a healthy lifestyle with balance.

Who Are You Doing This For?
by Gaby Sink

Who are you doing this for? Many have asked me why I do what I do, or how I have the drive to keep going. I have only one answer. I am doing this for me.

Growing up I was the thinnest and tallest in my class. All the way through high school I sat at about a buck twenty with not an ounce of fat on me. I played organized sports like volleyball and basketball through middle school and early high school. Having the body of an athlete, I didn't really care about anything.

My mom has always been my biggest supporter. She currently suffers from a variety of diseases I wish would just disappear. After she had me, she was diagnosed with hypothyroidism. Back then she was well controlled with medications. That was just the beginning though. The thyroid disease brought on a series of different things. Doctors were unable to control her thyroid hormone for a while, causing her to gain weight. When I was in early high school, she was diagnosed with SVT (supraventricular tachycardia) which caused her heart to race so fast she felt like she was having a heart attack, sending her to the ER several times. Later on she was also diagnosed with type two diabetes. That one really hit me hard..... This is my mother, the most beautiful woman I know - and she now suffers from one of the top killing diseases.

Shortly after she was diagnosed, I moved to Houston with my then boyfriend (now husband). After a year or so, I hadn't realized it, but I had gained a solid 40 pounds. I never got on the scale so I didn't realize it, not to mention my clothes still fit me - or so I thought. Ok, ok so my breasts were bigger and I was like - what is going on?

None of it hit me until I saw myself in a photo wearing a bikini -

rocking some serious saddlebags, big tummy and a chunky face.

My first reaction was "OH NO......"

My husband kind of let me know then - that I was getting chunky.

Chunky???!!! I was almost 50 pounds overweight, I don't want to say that I was fat, but at that moment, that is how I felt.

It didn't take me too long to realize, that wasn't me. What had I done? I was headed straight down the path of obesity, partying every weekend, eating fast food and drinking countless sodas throughout the day. I quickly made the change.

We joined a gym. I threw out all the crap food we had and we started from scratch.

I have not looked back. I found myself working out every day until I literally felt guilty if I missed a day. What a crazy feeling that was! About 6 months after I started, I had lost all the weight I had packed on. It was an amazing feeling to be in my usual weight range, where I was comfortable.

I started competing in 2011. I was officially addicted after my second show when I moved on to competing in the NPC, here in great state of Texas where bodybuilding and every division in it is extremely competitive. I myself am in the bikini division, where the judging gets weird. You really never know what the judges will be looking for. I have done eight shows and all my critiques have been different. I make it a point to come in at my very best.

Competing is unlike anything I ever imagined. Bikini girls see glitzy, glamorous and dangerously curvy. Going through getting the spray tan on which is extremely sticky and uncomfortable, to buying your custom bikini, getting beautified the morning of the show is what I love most! The experience of competing is amazing, especially when you are in a team. I am very happy to say I am on Team Bombshell, one of the top training teams in the world. They helped me bring my best to my last few shows.

Every girl needs a support group for this sort of thing, and being on a team gives you all the support you will ever need.

So after working out for 3-4 years, I no longer sit at 120 pounds. I gladly weigh 140 -145 pounds. That's right ladies, muscle weighs more than fat and over the past few years I've accumulated a good amount and I am very proud. I rarely look at the scale, I don't feel like I really need to anymore. I eat healthy and work out daily, which is what matters most to me.

Make time to make the lifestyle changes in your life. I know what its like to be busy. I have a full time job, I train every day, I do posing sessions with bikini girls, I train others, and I work for a supplement company on top of that. Oh did I mention I'm married? Yeah I know we can all agree that's like working a double.

This journey is mine. Whether I place at the shows, doesn't matter. It is a personal accomplishment. I want to be healthy I want to be around for my husband, future kids and my parents, especially my mom. I know she will need me someday and I want to be strong enough to aid to her.

So make it a point to really think about why you are doing this and who its for. It will keep you motivated.

This is your journey. Lead it to the finish line.

Gaby Sink
I'm an NPC bikini competitor and team bombshell athlete.

You Can Have Your Cake & Eat It Too
by Abi Christine Woodcock

The day my husband and I found out we were expecting our first child was a day full of joy, excitement, and uncertainty. During the months to follow I read every book I could find about what to expect in taking care of myself, and my new baby.

Prior to my pregnancy, I was not athletic and knew almost nothing about nutrition. I did a little cardio here and there and tried my best to eat healthy, or so I thought.

After we brought home our beautiful and healthy baby girl, life soon got back to normal and our same old routine was back on track. However, I very quickly realized that my body did not do the same! Before my daughter I had a little bump in the back, my belly was flat, and my legs were slender, but not anymore! I no longer had a butt, it had completely fallen flat, my belly had excess skin and a pooch, and the back of my legs were unrecognizable. I think anyone who has had a baby can identify with what I am talking about. I decided that I did not like what I saw in the mirror and I was not going to accept it as my fate. I was going to take control and not let the "I have kids" excuse take me down its path. I hired a trainer, started a new nutrition plan, and set goals for myself.

My very first goal was to compete in a fitness competition. I definitely had no idea what I had signed up for. It was difficult for me, the diet was completely foreign to anything I had ever done before, and the workouts were more strenuous than I ever expected. There were times during my competition prep when I wanted to quit but I knew I had to follow through and finish for "me". That night of my first competition, 7 months after I had my baby, I brought home my first trophy. The feeling of accomplishment and pride in what I had done was overwhelming. When it was all over I realized how much I liked the challenge and seeing the results of my hard work and dedication.

Since my first fitness competition I have competed in two additional shows and also picked up modeling along the way. I have learned a lot about myself through fitness and also gained a lot more confidence. I would never have believed you, if you told me 3 years ago, I would be where I am today in fitness. Honestly, I feel God has shown me more about myself in the past 3 years than I ever learned in the previous 25. I have become stronger, more assertive, and I feel I have finally found my true passion.

As time has gone on, and my passion for fitness has developed, there have been new and exciting opportunities, but with the opportunities has also come the lesson of learning balance. I receive emails every week asking how I manage to stay in shape while being a wife, mother, maintaining a career, modeling, and vigorously pursuing my passion of fitness. The answer is really very simple, I prioritize. Now actually putting that into action isn't all that simple.

Initially finding balance was a very big struggle for me. I had anxiety if I missed even one workout, my family was upset with me because I would pass on pizza night, my work was lacking my attention, and I was full of guilt. I knew I wasn't being fair to myself or my loved ones.

One of my favorite quotes is by Zig Ziglar, "I believe that being successful means having a balance of success stories across the many areas of your life. You can't truly be a success in your business life if your home life is in shambles.". So I took a step back and reevaluated my life. I began prioritizing and getting organized! I started making my meals ahead of time, so I can stay on track with my diet, I wake up earlier to fit in my cardio, and I weight train on Saturday and Sunday, because a few nights a week I have other obligations, and when my family wants to go out for our weekly pizza night, I am right there enjoying a few slices with them. I found my balance! Yes, there are times when things come up and put a snag in my schedule, but I move on and get right back on track!

I of course believe everyone has to find their own balance and that will vary depending on each individual, their priorities, and their lifestyle. I just want to show women, in particular mothers, that it is possible to pursue your passions, care for yourself and your family guilt free!

I can have my cake and eat it too.

Abi Christine Woodcock

I'm the wife to an amazingly supportive husband, the mother of a beautiful daughter, bikini competitor, fitness guru, and published model. I firmly believe you create your own path in this world.

From Frumpy Mom to Buff Mom
by Stephanie Woods

My name is Stephanie Woods and I am the owner of Stephanie. Fitness. I am an online personal trainer who is NASM certified. I'm married to a meathead who is my very best friend, Zack Woods, who owns and handprints his own fitness clothing called, Woods Strong. We have two rambunctious little boys, Ty and Dean, who are infatuated with big muscles and want nothing more than to get big like their dad. Together we live in Southeast Idaho and love nothing more than lifting weights, camping, razor riding, exploring ghost towns, eating Sushi, and supporting our kids in every sport possible.

I started Stephanie.Fitness on a whim back in April of 2011. I had a lot of family and friends that were asking me to share and post my recipes that I was starting to invent and come up with that helped me lose fat and build muscle. So, I started a small blog to share with my family and friends. Little did I know that Stephanie.Fitness would become so much more than that. I now offer online personal training, customized meal plans, fitness tips, product reviews, and more. But, there's more to me than just my website. Here is my story.....

I'm not going to begin to tell you how my childhood was other that than I never took health and fitness seriously. Like never. The thought of a skinny fit body never even crossed my mind. Of course, I was always into sports, but never looked at them like they were bettering my health. I did them because I enjoyed them and it was something to do after school. I did volleyball, basketball, and even at College I started a women's rugby team. I did sports because I enjoyed them. But, I still ate like a horse and was never taught the importance of proper diet and exercise. Even though I was active through high school and college, I still had hips the size of a

Buick and I was technically considered "skinny fat".

It wasn't till after having Dean, my youngest, that I really started to pay attention to what I ate and suddenly exercising became very important to me. During my two pregnancies, I never once worked out or cared about the way I ate. It wasn't important to me at the time. Yes, I was unhealthy and I was definitely unsatisfied by the way my body looked. I hated my hips, butt, and thighs the worse. I have always been very bottom heavy. I thought that God was playing mean tricks on me and decided to stick a skinny person's upper body on a fat ladies lower body. I was wearing size 10 pants at 5'2 and I was even trying my best to squeeze into those. After having Dean, I decided to make a change.

I eventually one day asked my husband for help. Zack has always been into bodybuilding, fitness and eating healthy even before I met him 11 years ago. But, his dedication and healthy eating habits never really rubbed off on me until after having our 2 children. I finally asked him for help. I still remember him pulling out a piece of paper and writing down a workout regimen for me that would target one to two body parts a day for five days a week. I had to ask him about proper form with my exercises as I was completely clueless to lifting weights. He was very helpful and guided me along. We never once went to the gym together. We couldn't. We had two small children and the gym he went to didn't have a Kids Klub. So, I signed up for Gold's Gym and he would write out my workouts for me and I would have to do them on my own. Trust me when I say, I felt very overwhelmed at first, but I was determined to look a certain way and I didn't care how long it took me to learn.

Little did Zack know that once he taught me about lifting weights, I would take off with his guidance and become a BEAST in the gym. I have to thank him almost every day, because if it wasn't for him helping me, I wouldn't be who I am today. He's my biggest motivator and supporter, but I don't think he realized he had unleashed a caged animal. I soaked up everything he taught me and then some. Within a few months I saw changes in my body and muscle definition that I had no idea even existed. Seeing my muscles pop in the gym mirror for the first time was the day I suddenly fell in love with lifting heavy weights and since then I've never looked back.

Over the last few years, I began to educate myself with Kinesiology, nutrition, and diet. Zack always knew about the weights and exercises, but it really wasn't until I started studying and researching about diet and food that our knowledge of a fit and healthy body truly grew. To this day, I'm constantly educating him and myself on diet and proper foods. And he still amazes me with the killer workouts that he can put together for me. Together we make a great team!

Back in 2011, I began training for my very first figure competition. I was so excited to start a new journey and I worked extremely hard and got so close to competing. But, I had to back out 2 days before my show due to a kidney infection from a severe case of strep throat that I had let go for far too long. That was stupid on my part and it really bummed me out that I got that close to a show and then never got to compete. I decided to put any competitions on hold and started focusing more on my career instead. I was working as a personal trainer at my local Gold's Gym at the time, but decided after a year it wasn't for me. I didn't like the management and unless you had a great clientele established you really didn't make a great income.

I hung onto my job at the gym as long as I could. In the last few months I began working closely with, Dr. Warren Willey, author of 'Better Than Steroids' and Board Certified Bariatric Physician. His CFO, Ace Call, contacted me and asked if I would be interested in working with Dr. Willey as his online personal trainer. I jumped at the chance to work with such a mastermind and we quickly became great friends. As soon as I began training people online for Dr. Willey, I came across a huge conflict with the gym I was currently working for and decided to quit in February of 2012 and began working full time with Dr. Willey.

I instantly fell in love with online training because it gave me twice as much accountability with my clients than I did when I actually trained them in the gym. With online training, I know exactly what workouts my clients are doing every week and I knew exactly what they were eating day in and day out. I never had that kind of "scheduling" with my gym clients. I worked for Dr. Willey for over a year and eventually the both of us decided it was time to part ways and go in different directions. Dr. Willey was starting a new program with hormone replacement therapy and I was starting to get too busy with my own personal website that I couldn't keep up with both.

I officially started training people online with my very own programs, systems, meal plan software and recipes in January of 2013 and I couldn't be happier. I learned a lot from Dr. Willey and I couldn't have gotten this far without him. But, going out on my own and really focusing on my career and my website has made a huge difference with my clientele and my responsibilities as an online trainer. I absolutely love my job and I love every single one of my clients. I'm here to help and motivate those who want to be fit and healthy like me.

Owning my own online business and trying to complete a recipe cookbook and e-book, while trying to run a household and raising 2 kids is hard. And on top of all that, I'm staying active and healthy. I'm busy just as much as the next person. Believe me when I say, I understand how hard it can be to take care of your kids, run them back and forth from school and sporting events, keep your house clean, run errands, do your finances, cook meals, and still have time for yourself and your husband.

It's hard! Especially, when you're also trying to squeeze in your workouts and stay on a good diet.

Here is the best advice I can give to all mom's out there:

1. Have a good support system. Whether it's your friends, your family, your husband, and/or your kids. If you don't have a good support system, it very hard to stay on track and feel confident in what you're doing.

2. Prep your meals ahead of time. If your meals are already cooked, chopped, and pre-portioned in the fridge, it is so much easier to just grab and go. The problem with people today is that they are constantly busy and heading to one thing to the next. Who has time to cook every single meal, every single day? I know I don't. So, choose one or two days a week to plan and prep all of your meals. If you don't have to think about your next meal or what to eat next because you've already planned it, you're more likely to stay on track with your nutrition and diet. And this can also apply to your significant other and children. Chop up veggies and fruit and leave it at eye level in the fridge for your kids. Keep their favorite yogurts and whole wheat products where they too can easily grab and go. Teach your children while their young. They watch us like hawks. So, if they see you eating healthy, they'll pick up on that as they get older.

3. Make time for the gym. For most people, they have a hard time just getting to the gym. Well, so do I. But, it's important enough to me that I MAKE time. If I start skipping days and not getting my exercise in every week, my body tends to get stiff, I get grouchy, and even moody. Exercising is a great stress reliever and I don't know one person that ever regretted going to the gym. Start managing your time better and schedule your gym time.

4. Stay consistent. This is the biggest misconception people have. If people don't see fast results, they tend to drift off their path instead of

staying consistent with their diet and exercise. There will be times during your journey that you won't see progress or results. You will need to be patient and push past those plateaus. Everyone deals with them, and whether you succeed or not will depend on how you well you handle your plateau. If your goal is to lose fat, you shouldn't treat it like a race. It took a long time to put that fat on and it's going to take time to take it all off. I typically like to see my clients lose about one pound per week. That's it. Any more than that, they're probably losing more muscle than they are fat.

5. Throw out your scale. Do not be constantly dwelling on numbers. Women especially seem to determine how the rest of their day is going to go by how their scale reads in the morning. If they don't like what they see, they're bummed out for the rest of the day and they think that they need to start eating salads and skip meals. WRONG! Screw what the scale says. If you're sticking to a good diet and proper calories and macros, you have no reason to doubt your progress. The human body fluctuates its weight by 1 to 6 lbs depending on the day or time of the month. Our bodies are consistently retaining water, flushing out water, increasing and decreasing blood flow, and so much more. Depending on your hormones for the day or what you ate the day before can make a huge impact on your body and water retention. Even the type of exercise the day before can make you retain water or expel it. Don't dwell on what your scale says. Your scale isn't going to tell you if you're retaining water. Your scale isn't going to tell you how much muscle mass you've put on. It's just telling you how much you weigh for the day. Focus more on how you feel, the extra energy you have now, and how your clothes fit.

6. Take progress pictures. Pictures can speak a thousand words. Our friends and family see us every day. We see ourselves in the mirror every day. Often times, we really don't see the progress we've made in a certain period of time until we go back to old pictures and compare our progress.

Pictures don't lie. Start keeping old photos so that you're constantly reminded of what you were before and to also remind yourself that you will never be that person again.

7. Lift weights and lift heavy. No, you will not get big muscles like a man. That is hormonally impossible unless you were to do some sort of hormone replacement therapy. Our bodies were made to work. So, make your muscles work. Shape them, define them, and exercise them. Lifting weights has been proven to improve arthritis, osteoporosis, and cardiovascular disease as well.

8. Cardio is over rated. I don't do a lot of cardio. I maybe do about 1 hour of cardio per week. That's it. And, the same goes for my clients. I don't have them doing ridiculous amounts of cardio. For the majority, I'm all about lifting heavy weights and focusing on diet. Ever since we were in elementary school we've been taught to run and sprint to stay healthy. Cardio is great to help with endurance and to help keep a healthy heart, but I don't like using it to lose fat. You will actually burn more calories by lifting weights than you would by doing cardio every day. When I go to the gym, I see the usual cardio bunnies that are doing 1 to 2 hours of cardio almost every day. I never see them incorporating weights. Yet, year after year, these people always look the same. They never change. Why is that? For one, they're all skinny fat. Too much cardio will actually make you lose muscle mass. You need muscles to burn calories and to shape your body. And two, most cardio crazy people are trying to burn "X" amount of calories because of what they ate the day before. It doesn't really work like that. Focus on your diet every day and incorporate weight training and you will see amazing results. You can't out train a diet. And you can't out run it either.

9. Set small goals. Big goals are great too, but doing a bunch of smaller ones to eventually equal one big one is more rewarding and satisfying to

the average person. Most people like to see things happen fast, so setting small goals that you can reach in a few weeks or even a few short months will not only help keep you motivated, but it will also keep you more focused and ready to move onto the next goal. If you set one big goal, it may almost be unreachable or take so long that you eventually lose interest. Setting goals that you can see in the near future or can reach in a short amount of time will help keep you on track.

10. Food is considered a drug. Many have become addicted to certain foods. Turning down sugary or fattening foods is going to happen almost on a daily basis. Our bodies constantly crave sugar and fat. But, as you start to weed those types of foods out, you'll notice you crave those foods less and less. But, turning down those foods are not going to be easy. You will have to practice will-power constantly. The more you practice will-power the better you will become at turning down certain foods. Until you can overcome your cravings or incorporate them only in moderation, you will never be truly satisfied with progress and goals. Don't give in. Keep pushing forward to maximize your results.

I train hard almost every day. I stick to a well-balanced diet every day. I'm constantly setting new goals. I have good days and bad days. I'm only human after all. Hitting the gym and sticking to a good diet should become habit to you one day. Just like taking a shower every day. If it's important enough to you, you will find time for it. You may have to sacrifice a few things to do it, but in the end it will always be worth it.

Practice will power, make time for the gym, prep your meals, set small goals, and ultimately focus on how you feel. Speaking of setting goals, my next goal is to complete a cookbook and e-book with my recipes for all to have in their homes. It has been something I've wanted to do for over 3 years now and hopefully I will have it finished by Summer 2014.

Stephanie Woods

I'm an online personal trainer & healthy recipe inventing Guru.

VOLUME V - MAKE A DIFFERENCE

Creating Love in Every Day
by Kyla Gagnon

There have been a few "moments" along the journey to my here and now, and knowing what a difference they've made for me, it seems like a good idea to share…

As a personal trainer, I've always loved feeling as though I have the opportunity to make a difference in the lives of others. I lost my mom and best friend shortly after my 20th birthday, definitely one of those "moments" I mentioned. Navigating my grief, feeling rather sorry for myself, and focusing a lot of energy on ME is something I'm so grateful to have been able to do, and the combination of that experience, my wonderful father, and learning to rely on myself has brought me where I am today.

You'd think with that under my belt, along with my career, I'd be all set to live a life of "moments" and make an impact on those around me. I suppose you'd be right…kind of. My career has been wonderful to me, I've had great clients, and along the way I was fortunate enough to meet a wonderful man who cared a great deal about me. How lucky was I?! I was fulfilled in my work, loved, fully supported emotionally, and had a hard-working, caring, beautiful man in my life. We traveled, spent quality time together, drank wine, and DID all of the things that I THOUGHT would fill me up, all of the things I believed would keep me fueled to give back to the world and leave a footprint of happiness and joy. I was living a lot of the "moments" that we aspire to live.

And I felt like I was so very far from who I was supposed to be.

It's a challenging thing to battle the mechanisms we all have operating our minds – we're doing what we're SUPPOSED to be doing, we're with who we're SUPPOSED to be with. I was living a life that included the so-called perfect man, who to this day, I couldn't say anything but kind and gracious things about. Social conditioning is a powerful tool and when I look back at the life I was leading, I was a working model of what all the "norms" around me have taught me to be.

So I did exactly what I was supposed to do, and what so many would have told me not to do. I left him. The possibility for the incredible, potentially enviable life with a wonderful person became a memory. What pushed me into this "moment"? The realization that before I could make a difference to my clients, to my friends, to my family, or to my partner, I had to make a difference to myself.

I'm not sure if there's supposed to be some grand epiphany that follows a life change like that, or if you're waiting for me to tell you that after being true to my feelings, I experienced growth that allowed me to realize that I belonged with that dear man. Nope. I mean, I experienced growth…it felt awful and uncomfortable and scary. And then it felt amazing and freeing. And it taught me that I was right to trust myself. I was right to listen to MY little voice and ignore all of the other big ones. I didn't belong with him. And that was okay.

Taking that leap and scaring myself to death was the best platform I could have ever imagined for giving myself the strength to have an impact in a real and authentic way. It empowered me to use my work not only to help people physically but as an outlet to show my love, and to provide loving emotions to multiple people everyday. It spread to my everyday interactions with strangers, to my relationships with my closest friends, and to the part of myself reserved for the one I love.

The journey has been a bumpy one since then, but I wouldn't change that for anything. My ability to be authentic in my life has reached a level I never imagined.

Don't get me wrong, I hit plenty of roadblocks still. I struggle to be open, I struggle to be vulnerable but if I learned anything from that incredibly difficult decision, its that the hardest things are often the most worthwhile. I know it's a cliché but it blows my mind how easily we detach from that notion, how we default into a safe mode that keeps us on a steady path, trying to avoid the turns and obstacles. Perhaps a break-up doesn't seem like that big of a deal to others but all I know is that the strength it took to end a relationship that everything in this world tells you is what you're supposed to want has pushed me into a future that I'm so excited about. And I'm excited because I can't help it, not because I think I'm supposed to be.

Part of this experience is feeling grateful, grateful for the gift of a life that allows for change. I now begin my day with a Gratitude and an Intention:

I am grateful to be alive today, life is beautiful...

My intention for this day is to create happiness with every person I am in contact with, clients, co-workers, strangers at the grocery store... people on the street.

By creating happiness in others, I too will feel happiness.

I'm far from perfect and I'm certainly not a monk and there are definitely mornings when this feels less than organic. But these mornings are the ones that count, the times when I sit up, take a big breath in, exhale it all out, feel whatever I am feeling inside today, and acknowledge that it will pass. These are the "moments" that I make a difference to myself, to ensure that I can always make a difference to others.

In health,

Real Talk Real Women

Kyla Gagnon

I'm the founder of Inside Out Fitness and BodyRipped.net, I'm madly in love with my career, as it provides me the opportunity to help guide others towards living their absolute best life possible.

Find Your Inspiration
by Jessica Jessie

When I look back on my high school years, not too many days stand out in particular. I was a very busy student balancing school with three sports: soccer, volleyball and basketball. I was also captain of the cheerleading squad but my Mom wouldn't let me do any of the activities that I loved if I didn't maintain good grades. That's why I'll never forget the day in tenth grade when my Mom let me skip school to meet my idol, the beautiful Cindy Crawford.

I always thought Cindy Crawford - and I still do - was the most beautiful woman on the planet. Not only was she pretty, but she was a successful businesswoman who carried herself with elegance, poise and style. She was everything I wanted to be as I was growing into a young woman. And when I finally met her during a book signing in McLean, Virginia I couldn't have been more thrilled. Getting a chance to talk to her for just a few minutes and see her impact on countless people inspired me to have a similar impact on what I'm truly passionate about, fitness.

The Oxford dictionary defines inspiration as the process of being mentally stimulated to do or feel something. Well just as Cindy Crawford inspired me as a 16-year-old girl I have tried to do the same. As a professional fitness competitor in the bikini division of the IFBB I want to be an example to women on how to attain a healthy, beautiful body. I'm very open about my training regimen and nutrition in blogs and social media so that women can see that if they work hard and have faith in the process they too can achieve their fitness goals.

Being a good example is very important if you want to inspire. Would you ever go to a hair stylist with bad hair? How about a dentist with bad teeth? That's why it's important to me to look my best whether I'm competing in the IFBB or simply working with my clients as a master personal trainer and certified nutritionist.

But being an example is not enough. If Cindy Crawford had been cold or mean to me when I met her I may not have chosen this path in life. Instead she actually took an interest in what I was doing and aspiring to be.

Listening matters. In fact it's one of the biggest factors in inspiring others. So many people I've come across have changed for the better because I simply took the time to listen. Before moving forward I need to find out what they are searching for, what fulfills them and what they love. Sometimes I have clients who prefer non-traditional exercises so I suggest activities like kickboxing. Other times I have clients who get bored easily so I constantly change their workout regimen. They key is establishing a connection, finding out what works for them and then continuing to inspire them through constant communication.

Encouragement is very important. We all have bad days. Becoming fit and healthy can be a challenge especially with our busy lives and fast food available at every corner. That's why letting people know it is okay to fail can be important. We all fail. But we shouldn't lament on these failures. Instead we need to keep moving forward. I constantly try to tell my clients that they can do it even when they have failed. Did Michael Jordan make all of his last second shots? No, but he kept shooting!

Even the fitness pros have days where we go off the deep end and binge. I have found that surrounding myself with people who are there for me is vital to my success. Hearing positive words from those that I care about brings out the best in me. That is why it's important to remind people of their strengths so they can believe in themselves even when they have stumbled.

Sharing my experiences can also serve as an inspiration. Though women may see my competition pictures which project a certain image, they may not know that I came from an obese family and that I struggled with my weight while working as a professional cheerleader for the Washington Redskins. It was during this period of my life that I had to teach myself how to live a healthy lifestyle. I became obsessed with learning everything about nutrition and exercise. Simply sharing these stories helps me connect with women by letting them know that they can change their lifestyles, that they can overcome rough periods during their lives, that they can overcome genetics and bad eating habits.

Although most women will never step on stage in a beauty pageant or fitness competition, I'm not that different than anybody else. So if I can do it, why can't you? That's my message of inspiration. You can do it! And no matter how hard it may seem and no matter how many times you may stumble, just keep moving forward. Keep chasing your dreams and going after your goals. You can do it!

It's crazy that it's been almost 17 years since I met Cindy Crawford. It seems like yesterday that I was watching her fitness videos in my basement and trying to style my hair just like she did. But the truth is though I've never met Cindy Crawford again, she's never left me. That's inspiration.

Jessica Jessie

I'm a master personal trainer and certified nutritionist who is passionate about fitness. I am also an IFBB fitness professional who has competed in two Miss Bikini Olympias and the Arnold Classic.

Making a Difference in the World
by Laura London

I work on a daily basis with people who know that they want to transform themselves physically and mentally. As human beings, we all have an innate sense that to be truly happy in life, we need to start that journey with a sense of worth in our own bodies and accomplishments. I've seen thousands of people take that first small step and then go on to become healthy and successful. The funny thing is that most of those people have also found that their personal development is still not enough to achieve true fulfillment and happiness in life. Most successful individuals find that despite their personal growth, they still have the overpowering need to "make a difference" in this world.

Individuals, who find the discipline and the self-motivation to change their own life, can still be overwhelmed by the task of making a difference in the world. We all feel like it would be an enormous task, and that anything that we can do as individuals, is too small and insignificant to make much of a difference. In fact, nothing could be further from the truth. It is not the size of the contribution to the world that matters, but rather your efforts and motivation in making that difference – even if it is just for one other person. The beloved Mother Teresa summed up this philosophy best with her famous quote, "If you can't feed a hundred people, then feed just one."

We should also seek to influence others to start doing things that make a difference, and the best way to convince other people is to lead by example. Make it a habit to do one small thing each day to make a difference in the world. Other people will notice. You don't need to do it in a flashy or self-serving way - just do it. Before long, the example that you set will begin to be followed by those around you and before you know it, you're one small drop of helping to make a difference, becomes a wave of people making a difference.

Begin to make a difference by doing anything to help someone that is in your power to do TODAY. Help someone without a car get to an appointment, and then help them find a way to get around whenever they need transportation. Offer to watch an overworked mother's child for a few hours every week, while she takes a personal time break. Make a small donation to a local charity that empowers people. All of these small things can get the process of "making a difference" started.

Once you get started, your daily personal example will empower others to make the same daily effort to change the world. To keep the process going, be generous in your praise and recognition of others who make a difference through their contributions. Help them blossom and grow in their efforts. By empowering other like-minded individuals, you can make a difference to the collective effort that is being made by all enlightened human beings. Let others know that you find value if their contributions.

"Thousands of candles can be lighted from a single candle, and the life of the candle will not be shortened. Happiness never decreases by being shared." – Buddha

The important thing in "making a difference" is to not focus too much on your own fulfillment in making your contributions, but instead focus on the happiness and power that you give to others. Share your riches and reveal to others the many riches that they have that may have been hidden to them. When you help other human beings unlock their potential, it enriches you as well. It's easy.

Finally, look to make a difference that is long term and permanent. The old proverb that if you give a man a fish, you feed him for a day, but if you teach a man to fish, you feed him for a lifetime, is so true. The good that we seek to do will make more of a difference when there's a long-lasting effect rather than a temporary effect. Too often, we help people in a way that only makes them feel more dependent and powerless. Try to help people in a way that it empowers them, by giving them the power to help themselves. Find solutions. Educate people. Teach them to help themselves and others.

So "make a difference" in this world, by first getting your own body, mind and life in shape. This first step gives you the energy, skills and motivation to help others. Then just take the time to lead the way by doing daily small exercises in kindness and charity. Next, follow up your individual efforts, by sincerely encouraging and acknowledging the contributions of others. Finally, look for ways to make a difference that are long lasting and that empower those who you help to also become "difference-makers". Before long you will have made a significant contribution to the world that will bring you a lifetime of blessings and happiness.

Laura London
I'm a board certified health counselor (AADP), weight loss & detox coach, speaker, fitness personality and mom of 3.

Never Give Up, Speak Out Loud
by Lindsey Meyer

As I stand on this cliff at the edge of the Earth, I stare into the sunset and gather my thoughts. I clear my head, take a deep breath, slowly let it out, and remember these words by Russell Simmons. "Be encouraged. Stay on your hustle. You can't fail until you quit." I committed myself to a theory of this sort as a young girl that was lost in a world of pain trying to find my way to happiness. My only hopes were to forget all the pain. This is where I suppose it all started for me; strength that is. Strength to make a promise to myself to overcome the obstacles I have been through and grow to be a powerful woman that achieves everything she dreams of. I think back today and I am overcome with emotion knowing how my faith and strength have turned me into the woman that I could only dream of at a young age. I only hope to help others fight through their obstacles and encourage them to strive for what they want based on my story.

For many years, I shut down that place inside myself that needed to rage, cry, and ask questions, and basically express myself. I still wake up at night in a cold sweat screaming after seeing visions of "him". "Him" is a monster to me that is now seen as inhumane in my eyes. However, now I am a woman who has recovered from what he did to me when I was younger. There were times when I thought everything was my fault, and after I was embarrassed to tell anyone what happened to me.

I will never forget the day that I knew I had to be strong and tell my mom and brother that my mom's significant other had been sexually abusing me. It took every ounce of strength to get the words out of my mouth to my brother first. It was like a bad dream that you want to open your eyes from, but you can't because it's a dream. However, I finally pushed the truth out to my brother one day in the middle of the kitchen. We cried at first, but we both quickly gained faith and strength to plan our next steps. What was happened needed to stop. Once I said it out loud finally, I knew that what he had been doing to me was wrong. We didn't hesitate in taking the next steps to tell our mom what was going on. In fact, we both told her that very night. I will always be thankful for how my mom reacted to such a horrible truth coming out. She didn't doubt me for a second, and immediately removed me from that monster.

There are many factors that affect monsters going to prison for sexual abuse. In my case, it involved being pulled out of school for questioning day after day. Unfortunately, after everything I poured out, there was not a confirmed conviction. At times I think it could be a result of me not providing or remembering enough. However, the true fact is that it is very hard to get conviction for sexual abuse. Eventually, it was time to recover and find my way to being normal. Normal to others meant seeing a therapist. However, it just wasn't for me. I told myself then that I would do everything I wanted to do in life, and I would never let this set me back. I began to learn that if you challenge yourself with something you know you could never do, you find that you can overcome anything. Frank Sinatra puts it simple, "the best revenge is massive success". I knew then that I would do whatever it took to succeed.

Over the years I grew into a very goal oriented and competitive person. You name a sport; I played it. I played soccer, basketball, softball, and I ran track. I giggle to myself now remembering old times and how I would shed tears over losing a game. However, competition and goals are embedded in my DNA. I am my own toughest critic. If the team did well, but my performance wasn't where I wanted it, I came crashing down on myself. This carried over with everything else like my schoolwork, and now with my career. I refuse to settle for just getting a job done.

Miriam Khalladi

I will always remember:

"The only way to do great work is to love what you do. If you haven't found it yet keep looking. Don't settle." - Steve Jobs

Entering my adult life I still stayed active playing in softball leagues, hiking, and running throughout the week. However, I did not understand heavy weight training and proper nutrition. I was always that person that said I would never give up my pizza, and I don't want heavy weights to make me bulky. However, I tried a consistent nutrition plan to have proper fuel while training for a race that is held in Austin each year. After a few weeks of training, I saw a huge difference and became excited. Once I conquered the race, I was quickly searching for a new fitness goal. I call this the beginning of my obsession. A friend of mine who competed in figure through Texas NPC (bodybuilding world) quickly gave me a nudge to try the sport. Without knowing anything at the time in regards to how long it would take to train for a show of this sort, I set my heart on the Texas Shredder. Most people train for a show over 13 weeks or more. However, I set my goal on the Shredder and it being 6 weeks away didn't have me backing down. Suddenly I was throwing heavy weight all over the gym, following perfect nutrition, and pushing my little heart out while running sprints. During this time, a particular quote from Ray Kroc is suitable. "Luck is dividend of sweat. The more you sweat, the luckier you get." I think I had sweated enough over six weeks to fill a lake! However, these wise words prove true. I was a very lucky girl when I stepped on stage 6 weeks later placing 3rd in my very first show.

Words cannot describe the feeling inside you when you step on stage for the first time. Throughout the process of training for a show there are times when you cry, times when you think you want to give up, times you are so sore you can barely walk, but you put one sore leg in front of the other to keep pushing. When you finally get on stage everything around you disappears. All you can think of is smile big because it is your time to shine like the biggest star. I didn't remember a single thing I did after I got off stage for my first time. Everything basically becomes a blur when you show your transformation. All of the time, hard work, sweat, tears, and changes turn you into a new person. They say you change the most in your twenties; well I became a completely different person.

After seeing what I was capable of, I became addicted to competing in Bikini Division for TX NPC. I competed over the next few years, did amazing, went to nationals to compete at USA's in Vegas, and started chasing a pro card for the sport. While training for nationals, I found that I was in the best shape of my life; yet so unhealthy. When training for a show, your body exerts everything out of it and you are usually competing at around 11-13% body fat. As a woman, it can be damaging to stay below 15% body fat for extended periods of time. Well, for me I stayed around 11% body fat for about 7 or 8 months. After nationals I tried to go back to being normal healthy, and I gained 20lbs. I was at an ultimate low depression in my life. None of my clothes fit, weight kept increasing, but I was eating very clean and working out hard. There was a time I vividly remember standing in my closet, breaking down into tears because not one pair of shorts would button. I couldn't understand what was happening to my body, but I knew something wasn't right. As a result, I began working with an amazing nutritionist who tested my hormones and confirmed that there was serious damage done to my body. He confirmed that no matter how perfect you eat, if your hormones aren't doing well you will not be able to lose weight. After turning to a variety of hormone medications and perfecting nutrition to eat triple the amount I used to eat, I was throwing around weight in the gym and slimming up again in no time at all. I was back to myself just in time for competing season to begin again. Naturally, I wanted to keep pushing to chase my dream of turning pro in the sport. However, my nutritionist warned me that he could get me there but it wasn't what my body needed. While he warned me I needed more time to eat more and do less cardio, I just thought about how I just wanted to get back on stage more than anything. Happiness was questionable at this point.

I began getting ready to compete in my practice show for nationals, but along the way I realized a very important lesson. I started competing to achieve ultimate health and fitness, and have a fun goal. However, over a couple of years I found that I really hadn't lived at all. I traded in my clear pair of competing heels for life and fun. I wasn't able to go out to eat with friends, I was too tired to attend any events at night, and I started missing very important times in my friends' lives. My fiancé was the most patient out of everyone; standing by my side supporting my every move. However, I could count on one hand the number of times we had gone out to dinner in the past year. I found fun alternatives for family and friend, but it was still very hard to take on a normal life with continually competing all season. I also had another hard battle with always trying to change my body to achieve the "bikini look" and get a pro card. As you remember I was an athlete to begin with. I naturally have very muscular legs. In bikini it's important to not be too muscular, too lean, and you must have a symmetrical body overall. I was critiqued at every show to bring down the muscle in my legs and increase my upper body in size. I am naturally built with very muscular legs, a log torso, and a petite upper body. This meant I was continually tearing down the muscle in my legs, piling on muscle in my upper body, and I had to hike the bottoms to my swimsuit up to give an illusion of shorter torso and longer legs. While prepping for my last competition I came to a reality check that I got "lost" in the sport and my obsession. What was originally a great fitness goal turned into an unhealthy obsession to change my body to what others wanted and cause unhealthy body images toward myself. One day I just really started thinking, "What are you trying to do?" When I couldn't answer that question without saying, "I want to become a pro", I knew I had to reevaluate my goals.

When I think back to the amazing feeling I had stepping on stage for my first show, I found that the feeling wasn't the same as it used to be. Competing had become a job in my life. When I wasn't in contest shape I became unhealthy with my body image and wouldn't even want to get into a swimsuit in front of others. The goal of being in the best shape of my life got lost. I realized I was alone with hormone issues, and unhealthy body insecurities. I made a choice that I would go out of competing with the same show I came in with. I had put in the hard work of training for a show, and I wasn't going to give up my goal just because I had a reality check. As a result, I competed at the TX Shredder once again. I placed 4th with the normal critiques that my legs were too muscular, and I wasn't symmetrical. The fact is that I can continue to decrease muscle in my legs and increase my upper body, but I had to realize that I just didn't have what it takes to turn pro in the sport. It's the same as any sport, not every minor league baseball player can play in the major leagues. I really enjoy the world of competing, and support anyone who has a show in mind for his or her big goal. However, I had to remove myself from that world in order to become healthy and be happy with me again. Once I realized that I got lost in obsession with turning pro instead of competing for fun, everything else was simple for my decisions. I became to discover a new even stronger me that was still in love with fitness, but learning to love myself as well.

One amazing thing that competing did help me with was modeling opportunities. When I was younger I always said I wanted to be a lawyer and a model. Funny girl. I was too short and muscular for typical modeling, and I didn't go to law school. However, I have made an amazing career as an education account executive and I am now a fitness model. The funny girl turns out to be a coincidental story in the end.

I love being a fitness model because it reminds me how strong and beautiful I am. It is better to balance with normal life, but it keeps me on track consistently with my fitness goals. I find the same thrill in meeting new people and jumping in front of a camera, as I did stepping on stage. Plus I am also still a bikini coach for girls that are looking to compete. I teach them the importance of having a nutritionist and resting your body. I can't say I am 100% healthy with hormone damage and body image issues, but I have greatly improved. I am enjoying the discovery of a new me once again.

I like to revisit that cliff every now and again to gather my thoughts and ground myself with my goals. I know that I have been through many horrific issues in my life, but I know I will never let those things hold me back. I promised myself I would be a strong woman. That is something I am very proud to be today. As Michael Jordan says, "If you're trying to achieve, there will be roadblocks. I've had them; everybody has had them. But obstacles don't have to stop you. If you run into a wall, don't turn around and give up. Figure out how to climb it, go through it, or work around it."

Lindsey Meyer

I'm just a small town girl from MO that lives for fitness, competition & adventure. I balance fitness modeling, a full time career, and a family all at once. I thank God everyday for making me a strong fighter in life.

Finding Fulfillment by Sharing Energy
by Heather Nicholds

In order for me to be totally fulfilled by my work, I need to contribute to something beyond myself. There's a balance, of course. I need to take care of myself first in order to be able to give to others, but I don't find true inspiration doing things just for me. I see that even in everyday things like making dinner. If it's just dinner for me, it usually winds up being some raw vegetables tossed with beans. When I make dinner for someone else, I have a reason to put more effort into making something more involved, like veggie burgers with sweet potato fries and avocado dip.

My work also inspires me to make more interesting meals, because filming and posting recipes is like cooking for someone else. Although it may seem very practical and straightforward, the work I do in creating recipes and meal plans is my way of connecting with people. When you're able to connect with people who share your values, you can mutually inspire each other. What excites me about my work is not simply sharing recipes. What excites me is that I can contribute to the health and energy of someone else. The pathway I'm using is through healthy food, but my vision is to create positive energy cycles.

Over the years, I've learned that when I share my energy, not only do I give someone a boost, but just seeing them get that lift, and knowing that I played some small part in it, energizes me in return.. That's what I call a positive energy cycle – where the energy just keeps feeding itself and spiraling upward, as opposed to the downward spirals we usually think about. When we share energy with others, it can grow and magnify.

There are usually certain people in your life who feed that energy particularly well. I try to make it a priority to connect with those people often, and to build and maintain a strong connection. That is so much more valuable to me than anything else in my life because it creates the magic in any specific situation. When you have that kind of connection, you can make the most ordinary event – like going for a bike ride – into a special occasion.

As wonderful as some jobs sound, there are always some tasks and days that can get pretty boring. I spend a lot of time on my computer, replying to comments and questions or working on spreadsheets to get the right balance in a meal plan. The light that motivates me to do those tedious parts of my work is that overall vision of contributing more positive energy in the world. The really inspiring part is not only thinking about the people I connect with directly, but all the people they can inspire in their lives. When I look at life in that way, it's both humbling and empowering. Each one of us has an impact on everyone around us. The important part is how we choose to use that power.

My moments of feeling totally fulfilled from my work come when I get a note from a client or a viewer who says that they've started to actually enjoy making (and eating!) healthy food, and that it is inspiring them to enjoy more in their life. Whether they've found energy to play with their grandchildren, or appreciate being able to go for a walk in the sunshine, or just a sense of feeling good about themselves because of the nourishment they're giving themselves for the first time – these are the messages which inspire me to do more in my work and my life.

Too often in our busy lives, we neglect taking care of ourselves. When we remember to nourish ourselves, what tends to happen is that we remember to take care of other aspects of ourselves and our lives. What I've noticed is that no matter where someone starts – whether with nutrition or exercise or relationships or activities – the fundamental message is to respect and love oneself.

When you become aware of and remember to respect yourself, that awareness starts to spread into all aspects of your life. It also naturally spreads outward, so you become more aware of the people around you and then more aware of the whole ecosystem of life around all of us. It's especially rewarding to spread energy outward when you start to see those positive energy cycles boosting you right back.

It can be as simple as smiling at someone when you walk by each other on the street. Do you ever notice how when someone smiles back at you, you feel instantly happy? Even that little connection, that little bit of shared energy, can be so powerful. I love knowing that the more of myself I put out into the world, the more energy and inspiration I can spread and also receive. In a world where we're becoming more and more aware of the earth's dwindling resources, it's so refreshing to focus on an aspect of humanity that has infinite possibilities.

Heather Nicholds
I'm a holistic nutritionist, showing you how to have fun making simple, fast, delicious and nutritious meals.

Inspire People
by Valerie Solomon

What an honor it is to write a chapter for a book by inspiring women. To be honest with you, I have sat down several times to write this chapter and just stared at a blank page. How do I pick 750 - 1500 words from my life and my crazy mind to share with you? How did I get to this point?! How was I included in this book? Why is my life inspiring? I am nothing out of the ordinary...

Maybe you are having these same thoughts about yourself as you read through this book. Do you see yourself as an inspiration? I am willing to bet that you are much like me and that you do not. It is hard for us to see ourselves from the outside looking in. We know little details about ourselves that others do not. We know we have our own struggles, doubts, weaknesses, and challenges. We feel we are ordinary.

People relate to others like themselves... ordinary people. Wouldn't you love to hear how a woman just like yourself managed to lose 50lbs, run a marathon, start a business, climb a mountain, etc.? Many times we are inspired and motivated when we see someone in our own shoes showing us the way. It is often easier to take the first steps, if someone has walked the path ahead of you. Maybe it is a friend, a sister, or a social media personality that is similar to you. Ordinary people doing extraordinary things inspire.

So, I ask you this question: Are you missing an opportunity to inspire?

Are there people in your life that could benefit greatly if you were the first to make a move? We can choose to continue to keep to ourselves, keeping our talents, passions, and dreams a secret. Or we can take a chance and let the world know. The only reason that I am a part of this book is that I took a little leap of faith on a whim and started sharing my passion and talent on social media. I know I am ordinary…. Except I have this deep burning desire to be better, to do more, and to challenge myself. And that, it seems, is a talent and inspiration in itself.

After just over 2 years as "Busy Mom Gets Fit", I can honestly say that the best compliment is "You inspire people." What a gratifying feeling to know that what comes easy to me: fitness, motivation, busy-mom-life, is helpful to others in a big way.

"What comes easy to me…" Is that the key to it all?

Are you wondering what it is that you should be sharing? What comes easy? I firmly believe that we were each given talents, dreams, and passions for a reason. What is it burning inside of you to get out? What do you have to share with the world?

Here are a few steps that may help you step out on a limb to being an inspiration to those in your life:

1. Say you will

The first step to making a change or working towards a goal is committing. I you feel strongly and passionately about reaching a goal or making a change, just say you will do it. Write it down. Own it. You can figure out the details later.

2. Eliminate excuses

Start thinking through how you will accomplish your goal by pin pointing the hurdles in your way. Once you see clearly what has held you back in the past, you can start to find ways to make it happen. Maybe childcare has been an issue. Solve it. Maybe you feel like you do not have enough time. Cut something else out. For every challenge, there is a way to get through it. You have to do that for yourself and for those that need you to be an example for how it is done.

3. Realize and use your talents

So often we do not even realize our own strengths and talents. It comes easy to us and we don't realize that that is unique! What are people urging you to do? Or what are you complimented on? Listen to them! Sometimes a little shove from a good friend is just what we need to reach our potential.

The fact that you are reading this book is a pretty good indication that you are interested in growing and reaching your full potential. I hope you will share your journey with the world. I hope I read a chapter by you one day. Inspire people.

Valerie Solomon

I'm the founder of "Busy Mom Gets Fit". Busy mom of 4 boys, Army wife, figure competitor... living fit despite my crazy life.

About Miriam Khalladi

When a 20-something law student from Amsterdam stumbled into the fitness industry, she did not yet realize how that would change her life, and the lives of women across the globe.

"I just wanted to help women. Give back. Do good. Make a difference." says Miriam Khalladi.

Not considering herself an authority in the field, she set out to learn from and share the stories and life changing lessons of some of the most renowned experts and thought leaders in the field of health and fitness, while at the same time overcoming her own shyness.

On a mission to inspire women across the globe to live healthier, happier lives, she has interviewed top fitness competitors, elite trainers, Olympic gold medalists, martial arts champions and leading PhD's – focusing on their knowledge rather than their physical appearance.

Now, over 100 episodes of her web-TV show "Real Talk. Real Women." later – Miriam Khalladi is one of the most promising Media Entrepreneurs in the area of health and fitness.

> *"It's an amazing feeling to know that you're touching lives. Not even mentioning the incredible impact it has had on my own life. These women are all amazing."*

Miriam currently lives in Amsterdam, the Netherlands.
For more information or to reach out to Miriam,
please visit www.realtalkrealwomen.net

There's More!

Congratulations, you made it to the end of the book! First of all, I'd love to know what you think. What was your favorite chapter? Did you have an "a-ha" moment, or maybe several? Drop me a note via www.realtalkrealwomen.net and let me know!

Also, I'd like to invite you to our VIP newsletter. In it, you'll find the latest interviews with leading women in the industry, featured expert content and much, much more…!

I send it out about once a week, and it's completely free. You can join the list at www.rtrw.me/viplist/

Thank you once again for your support and make sure to find me on Facebook (www.facebook.com/miriamkhalladi) or Twitter (www.twitter.com/miriamkhalladi) and come say Hi!

Lots of love from Amsterdam,
Miriam

Write & Publish Your Own Book?

Did you know that more than 80% of people say they want to write a book, but less than 1% do? We get it, it's not easy.

That's why, from time to time we open up opportunities for lifechangers to come work with us. The thing is, we're nothing like a traditional publisher.

We coach you 1:1 through the writing process, from the structure of the book all the way through the final rounds of proofreading. We help you make the book look amazing, both on the inside and on the outside. And finally, we provide world class marketing support so that your book actually gets bought and read. Oh, and you can keep all the revenue.

If you've dedicated your life to helping others live happier, healthier lives - this is your chance to put a checkmark next to "publish my own book" on your bucket list.

Heard enough?

Contact us directly at publish@lifechange.io for more information.

www.ingramcontent.com/pod-product-compliance
Lightning Source LLC
Chambersburg PA
CBHW071257110426
42743CB00042B/1077